Student Workbook for

FUNCTIONAL ANATOMY

Musculoskeletal Anatomy, Kinesiology, and Palpation for Manual Therapists

Christy Cael   BS, ATC, CSS, LMP, ABMP

 Wolters Kluwer | Lippincott Williams & Wilkins
Health
Philadelphia • Baltimore • New York • London
Buenos Aires • Hong Kong • Sydney • Tokyo

Acquisitions Edition: Kelley Squazzo
Development Editor: Laura Bonazzoli
Product Manager: Erin M. Cosyn
Marketing Manager: Shauna Kelley
Manufacturing Manager: Margie Orzech
Design Coordinator: Doug Smock
Production Services: Aptara, Inc.

1 2 3 4 5 6 7 8 9

Contents

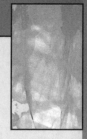

Introduction to the
Human Body

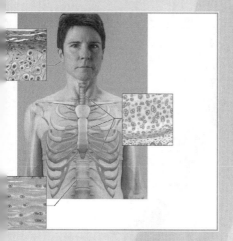

Anatomists and clinicians use a common language and universally accepted points of reference. The activities in this chapter are designed to help you become familiar with these tools.

IDENTIFY REGIONS AND DIRECTIONS

The following activities will help you more effectively communicate about the body, how it is organized, where structures are located, and how it moves.

INSTRUCTIONS. On the figures below, label the body region to which each line points.

List of Regional Terms

antebrachial
axillary
brachial
buccal
carpal
coxal
cranial
digital (use
    twice)
dorsal
facial
femoral
inguinal
mental
nasal
oral
orbital
patellar
pectoral
pubic
sternal
tarsal
tibial
umbilical

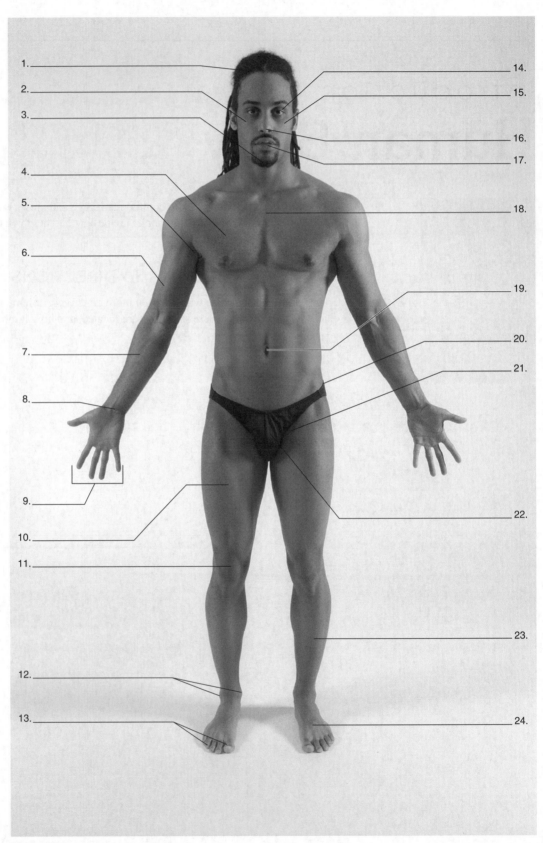

1. _____
2. _____
3. _____
4. _____
5. _____
6. _____
7. _____
8. _____
9. _____
10. _____
11. _____
12. _____
13. _____
14. _____
15. _____
16. _____
17. _____
18. _____
19. _____
20. _____
21. _____
22. _____
23. _____
24. _____

Figure 1.1

List of Regional Terms

acromial
calcaneal
cephalic
cervical
dorsal
gluteal
occipital
olecranal
plantar
popliteal
sacral
scapular
sural
vertebral

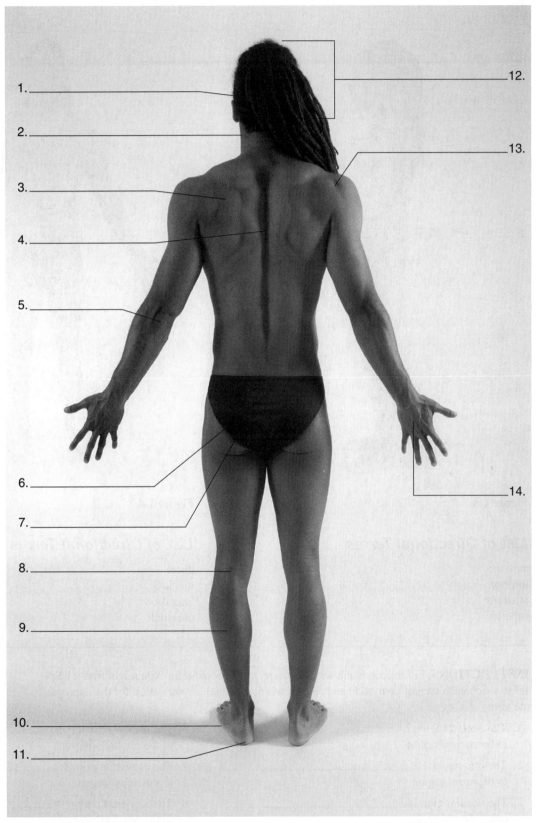

1.
2.
3.
4.
5.
6.
7.
8.
9.
10.
11.
12.
13.
14.

Figure 1.2

INSTRUCTIONS. Identify each relative direction in the pictures below by writing the appropriate term beside the arrow.

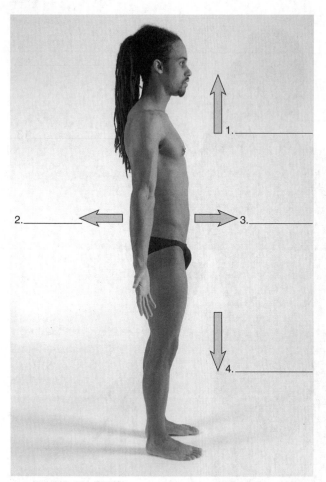

Figure 1.3

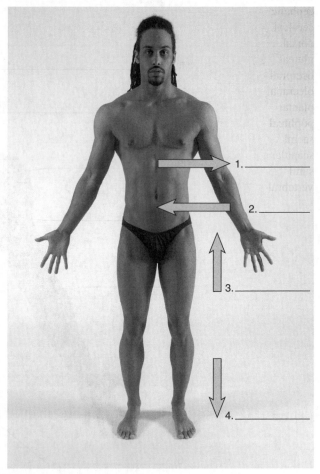

Figure 1.4

List of Directional Terms

anterior
inferior
posterior
superior

List of Directional Terms

distal
medial
lateral
proximal

INSTRUCTIONS. Fill in each blank with the correct directional term. You might find it helpful to touch each area of your body and say the words out loud as you search for the appropriate term.

1. The *orbital* region is _____ to the *mental* region.

2. The *otic* region is _____ to the *nasal* region.

3. The *nasal* region is _____ to the *frontal* region.

4. The *manual* region is _____ to the *cubital* region.

5. The *abdominal* region is _____ to the *vertebral* region.

6. The *occipital* region is _____ to the *popliteal* region.

7. The *cranial* region is _____ to the *tarsal* region.

8. The *acromial* region is _____ to the *brachial* region.

9. The *sternal* region is _____ to the *pectoral* region.

10. The *sacral* region is _____ to the *pubic* region.

IDENTIFY PLANES AND MOVEMENTS

INSTRUCTIONS. Fill in each blank with the correct term.

1. At the start of a card game, you cut the deck of cards by taking half the deck from the top. You have cut the deck in the _____ plane.

2. You are making a banana split. You peel the banana, then cut it lengthwise from top to bottom, separating it into a right and left side. You have cut the banana in the _____ plane.

3. You are building a campfire. You take a dead tree branch and snap it in two. You have snapped the branch along the _____ plane.

4. A child making a snow angel _____ and _____ the arms and legs.

5. In kicking a ball, a player _____ and _____ the knee.

6. In scanning the horizon, a sailor _____ the head.

IDENTIFY TISSUES AND THEIR FUNCTIONS

Now that you've practiced the language of anatomy, it's time to dive into specific structures of the human body! Let's begin with tissues.

INSTRUCTIONS. Each image depicts one of the four types of tissue found in the human body. Beneath each, identify which type of tissue is depicted: *epithelial, connective, muscle,* or *nervous.*

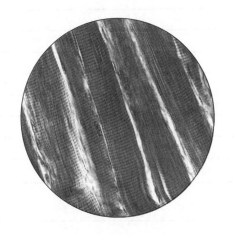

1. _____

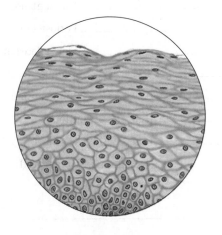

2. _____

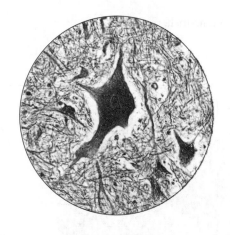

3. _____

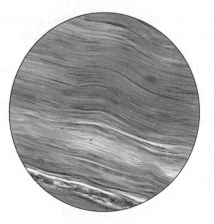

4. _____

Figure 1.5

INSTRUCTIONS. Match each of the four types of tissue with the correct function.

1. _____ Epithelial   A. Supports other tissues, transports nutrients and wastes, protects against outside invaders, and stores energy

2. _____ Connective   B. Protects, absorbs, filters, and secretes substances in the body

3. _____ Muscle   C. Receives and responds to stimulus via electrical impulses

4. _____ Nervous   D. Allows internal and external movement

INSTRUCTIONS. Identify whether each of the following is an example of *epithelial, connective, muscle,* or *nervous* tissue by filling in the answer blank with the appropriate term.

_____ Fat

_____ Sweat glands

_____ Periosteum

_____ Skin surface (epidermis)

_____ Tongue

_____ Joint capsule

_____ Blood

_____ Cartilage

_____ Spinal cord

DESCRIBE STRUCTURES INVOLVED IN MOVEMENT

Now let's explore the structure, function, and location of structures involved in movement.

INSTRUCTIONS. On the lines provided for each structure, list two functions and two properties that help you identify or differentiate the structure from other structures during palpation.

Bone _____

_____

_____

_____

Ligament _____

_____

_____

_____

Muscle _____

_____

_____

_____

Tendon _____

_____

_____

_____

Fascia _____

_____

_____

_____

IDENTIFY SPECIAL STRUCTURES

It's time to review the role of several complementary structures that protect, nourish, regulate, and support the function of those mechanically creating movement.

INSTRUCTIONS. Label each image with the items listed.

List of Structures

Blood vessels
Dermis
Epidermis
Hair shaft
Hypodermis
Muscle
Nerve

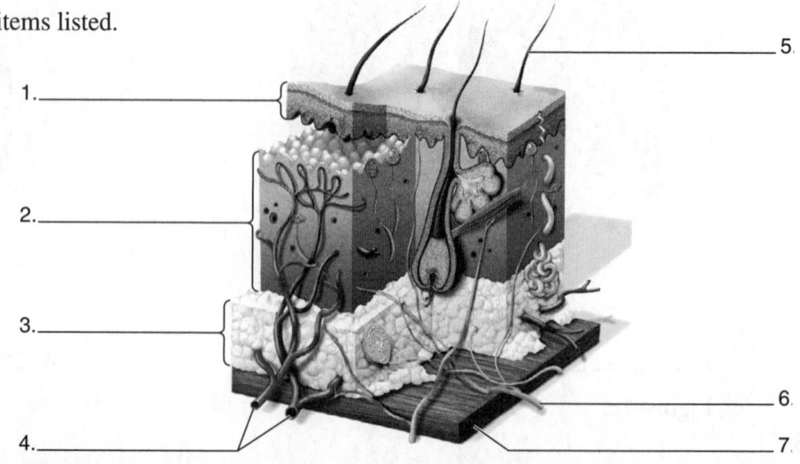

1. _____

2. _____

3. _____

4. _____

5. _____

6. _____

7. _____

Figure 1.6

List of Structures

Abdominal aorta
Anterior tibial artery
Anterior tibial vein
Axillary artery
Axillary vein
Brachial artery
Brachial vein
Brachiocephalic artery
Cephalic vein
Common carotid artery
Common iliac artery
Common iliac vein
External jugular vein
Femoral artery
Femoral vein
Great saphenous vein
Heart
Inferior vena cava
Popliteal artery
Popliteal vein
Posterior tibial artery
Radial artery
Subclavian artery
Subclavian vein
Superior vena cava
Ulnar artery

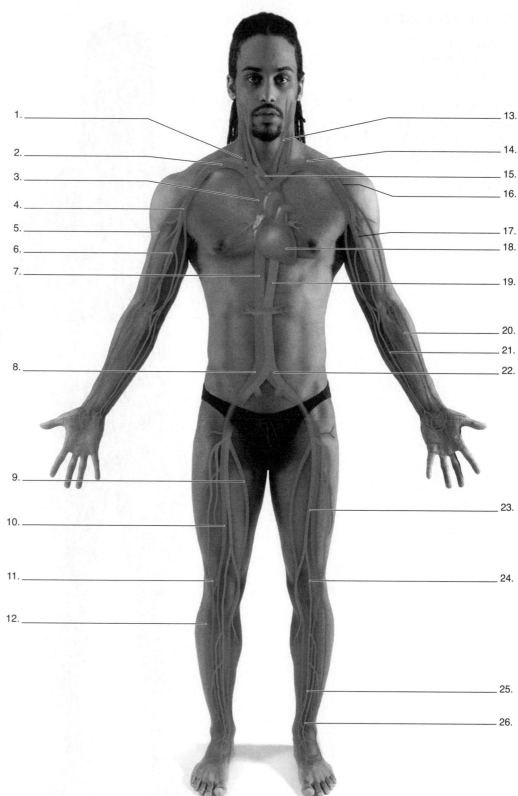

Figure 1.7

List of Structures

Axillary lymph nodes
Cervical lymph nodes
Cisterna chyli
Heart
Iliac lymph nodes
Inguinal lymph nodes
Popliteal lymph nodes
Right lymphatic duct
Spleen
Thoracic duct
Thymus

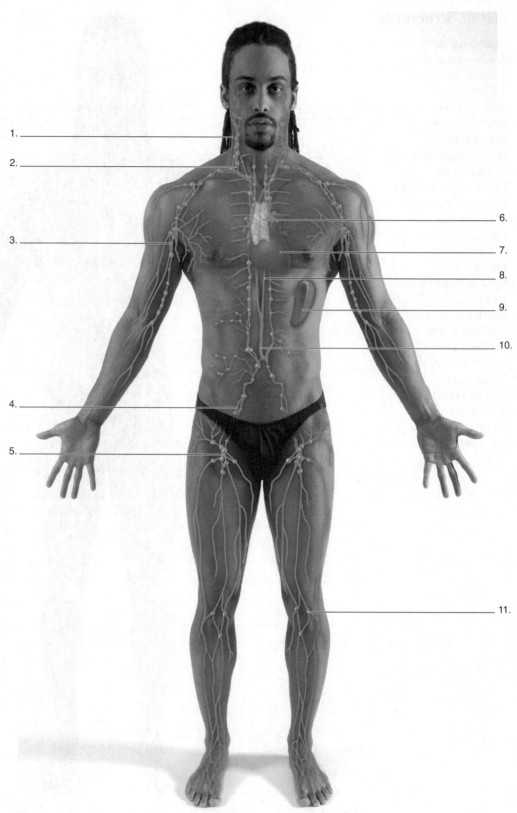

1. _____

2. _____

3. _____

4. _____

5. _____

6. _____

7. _____

8. _____

9. _____

10. _____

11. _____

Figure 1.8

List of Structures

Brachial plexus
Brain
Cerebellum
Cervical plexus
Common peroneal nerve
Intercostal nerves
Lateral femoral
  cutaneous nerve
Lumbar plexus
Median nerve
Musculocutaneous
  nerve
Radial nerve
Sacral plexus
Saphenous nerve
Sciatic nerve
Spinal cord
Tibial nerve
Ulnar nerve

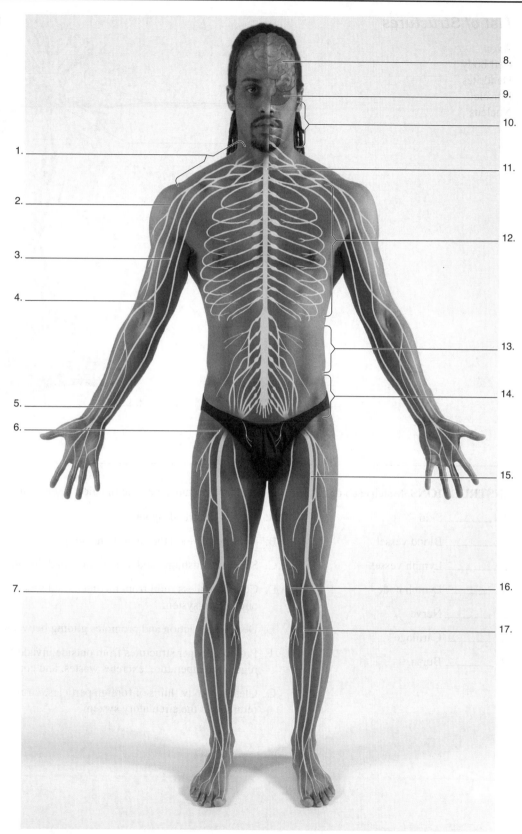

Figure 1.9

List of Structures

Axon
Cell body
Dendrites
Muscle
Nucleus

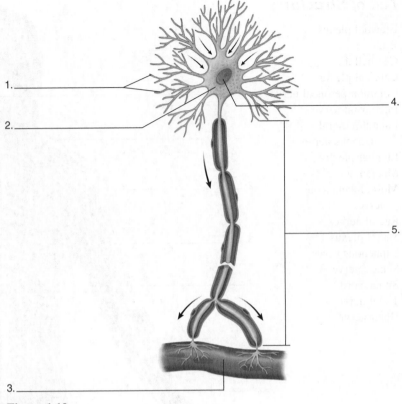

Figure 1.10

INSTRUCTIONS. Match each of the following special structures with the function it serves in the human body.

1. _____ Skin

2. _____ Blood vessel

3. _____ Lymph vessel

4. _____ Lymph node

5. _____ Nerve

6. _____ Cartilage

7. _____ Bursa

A. Carries electrical signals

B. Transports blood throughout the body

C. Supports, cushions, reduces friction, and distributes force at joints

D. Collects excess fluid from the interstitial space and returns it to the circulatory system

E. Decreases friction and promotes gliding between structures of movement

F. Protects deeper structures from outside invaders and radiation, helps regulate temperature, excretes wastes, and contributes to sensation of touch

G. Cleanses body fluids of foreign particles, viruses, and bacteria before it is returned to the circulatory system

WORD CHALLENGE

This final exercise checks your recall of terms and concepts introduced throughout the chapter.

INSTRUCTIONS. Unscramble each word and match it to its description.

1. ipifuscreal _____
2. acadul _____
3. milui _____
4. eastnail _____
5. tomosh _____
6. iltengam _____
7. meade _____
8. usrab _____
9. sixa _____
10. nilidem _____

A. Protein in branched, wavy fibers that confer resiliency to tissue
B. Fibrous structure that connects bones
C. Small, flat sac containing synovial fluid
D. Term for the center of the body
E. Type of muscle present in the walls of hollow organs
F. Closer to the surface of the body
G. A pivot point
H. Synonym for inferior
I. Abnormal accumulation of interstitial fluid
J. Example of a flat bone

Osteology and Arthrology

2

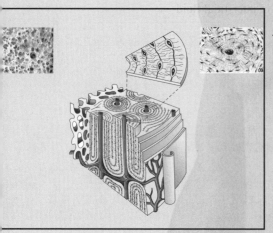

The activities in this chapter will help you develop your knowledge of bones and joints. You will relate the structure and shape of bones to the various roles they play in the human body.

IDENTIFY THE FUNCTIONS OF BONE

Why do we need bones? What purpose do they serve in the human body? Complete the following activity and discover the answers!

INSTRUCTIONS. In the space provided, list the four functions of bone. A clue is provided for each function.

1. _____ Clue: Think of the rib cage or skull.

2. _____ Clue: In this role, bones act as levers.

3. _____ Clue: This happens in bone marrow.

4. _____ Clue: Think of bones as nutrient banks.

IDENTIFY STRUCTURES IN BONE TISSUE

Bone cells are constantly at work deconstructing and constructing bone tissue. The following activities will help you learn the microscopic structures of bone tissue and their functions.

INSTRUCTIONS. Label the following image of bone tissue with the structures listed:

List of Structures

Canaliculi
Compact bone
Concentric lamellae
Haversian canal
  (appears twice)
Lacuna
Osteocyte
Osteon
Periosteum
Spongy bone
Volkmann canal

1._____

2._____

3._____

4._____

5._____

6._____

7._____

8._____

9._____

10._____

11._____

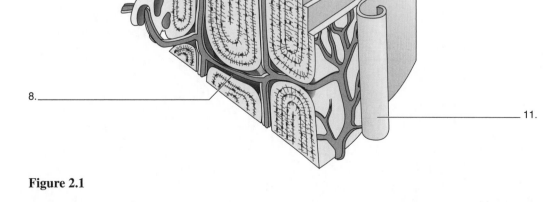

Figure 2.1

INSTRUCTIONS. Match each of the following structures of bone with the correct function by placing the letter in the space provided.

1. _____ Canaliculi
2. _____ Haversian canal
3. _____ Lacuna
4. _____ Lamella
5. _____ Osteocyte
6. _____ Osteon
7. _____ Periosteum
8. _____ Volkmann canal

A. Main opening for blood vessels and nerves in compact bone

B. Surrounds the outside of a bone and provides nourishment and protection

C. House microscopic blood vessels and nerves that serve outlying osteocytes

D. Cavity in compact bone that houses osteocytes

E. Functional unit of bone tissue, containing a Haversian canal and several lamellae

F. Concentric circles of lacunae that surround a Haversian canal

G. Pathways for blood vessels and nerves that run perpendicular to the Haversian canals and connect the bone surface to interior structures

H. Bone cells that regulate the constant remodeling of bone tissue

IDENTIFY BONES OF THE HUMAN SKELETON

INSTRUCTIONS. Label each of the bones in the following images by writing the name of the bone next to the correct leader line. Then, color the bones of the *axial* and *appendicular skeleton* using two different colors.

List of Bones

Carpals
Clavicle
Coccyx
Cranium
Face
Femur
Fibula
Hip (coxal) bone

Humerus
Metacarpals
Metatarsals
Patella
Phalanges (use twice)
Radius
Ribs

Sacrum
Scapula
Sternum
Tarsals
Tibia
Ulna
Vertebrae

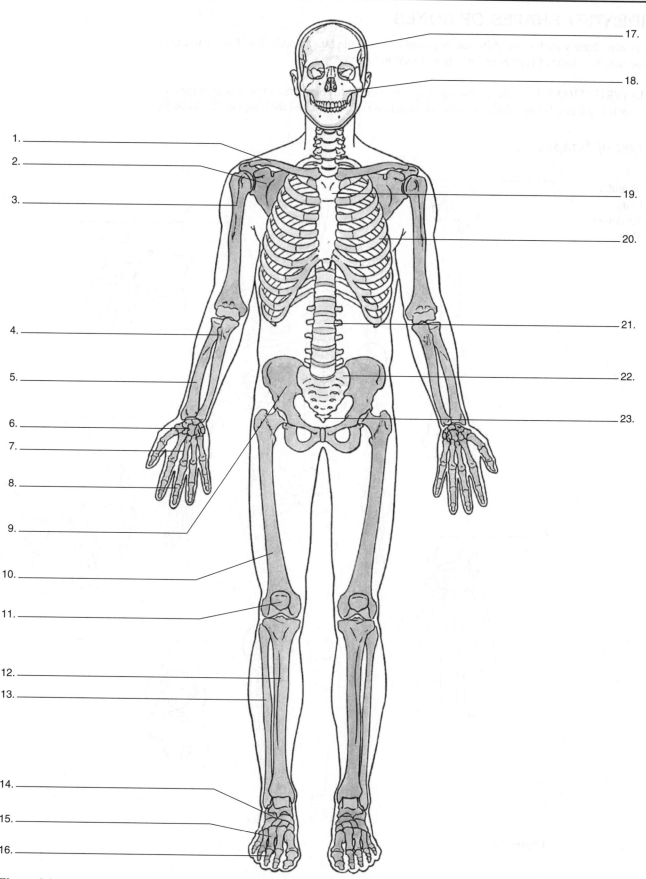

Figure 2.2

IDENTIFY SHAPES OF BONES

As you identify each of the different shapes of bones in the human body, see if you can imagine how the shape of each bone reflects its function.

INSTRUCTIONS. Label the following picture by writing the bone shape name next to the corresponding letter. Using a different color for each bone shape, color all the bones of the skeleton.

List of Shapes

Flat
Irregular
Long
Sesamoid
Short

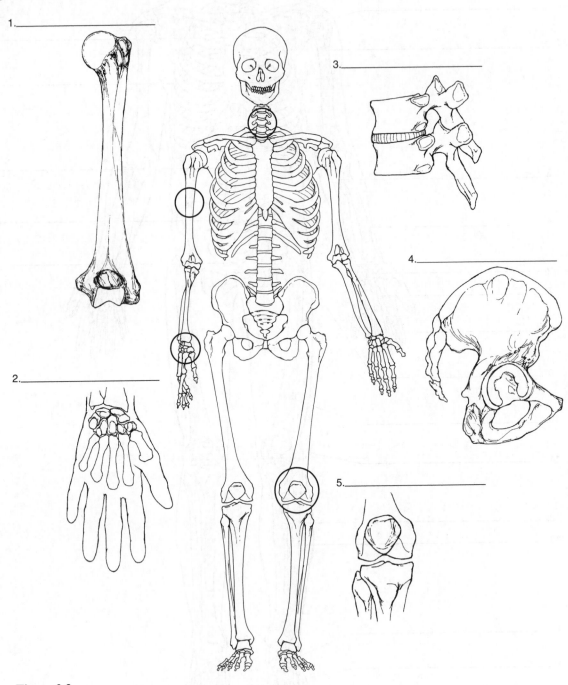

1._____

2._____

3._____

4._____

5._____

Figure 2.3

CLASSIFY BONY LANDMARKS

Bumps, ridges, holes, and depressions each serve a unique purpose for bone health and function. The following activities explore the functions and names of the different bony landmarks.

INSTRUCTIONS. Briefly describe the function of each of the following types of bony landmark:

1. Depression _____

_____

2. Opening _____

_____

3. Projection _____

_____

4. Attachment site _____

_____

INSTRUCTIONS. Identify the type of bony landmark (*depression, opening, projection,* or *attachment site*) by placing a D, O, P, or A in the space provided.

1. _____ Condyle
2. _____ Crest
3. _____ Epicondyle
4. _____ Facet
5. _____ Fissure
6. _____ Foramen
7. _____ Fossa
8. _____ Groove
9. _____ Head
10. _____ Line
11. _____ Meatus
12. _____ Process
13. _____ Ramus
14. _____ Ridge
15. _____ Sinus
16. _____ Spine
17. _____ Trochanter
18. _____ Tubercle
19. _____ Tuberosity

IDENTIFY JOINTS

Use the following activities to discover how bones fit together to form joints and rules for naming joints in the human body.

INSTRUCTIONS. State the basic rule for naming joints.

Joints are named according to _____ .

Name the joint formed by the articulation of the humerus with the ulna.

_____

How is the naming rule modified if one bone forms multiple joints?

_____

Name the joint formed by the articulation of the glenoid fossa of the scapula with the humerus.

_____

INSTRUCTIONS. In the space provided, identify the joint type as fibrous, cartilaginous, or synovial for each of the following:

_____ Acromioclavicular

_____ Carpometacarpal

_____ Costochondral

_____ Coxal

_____ Glenohumeral

_____ Humeroulnar

_____ Intercarpal

_____ Interphalangeal

_____ Intervertebral

_____ Patellofemoral

_____ Pubic symphysis

_____ Radiocarpal

_____ Radioulnar (proximal and distal)

_____ Sacroiliac

_____ Sagittal suture

_____ Sternoclavicular

_____ Talocrural

_____ Tibiofemoral

_____ Tibiofibular (proximal and distal)

CLASSIFY AND DESCRIBE SYNOVIAL JOINTS

Synovial joints typically have the most movement. Why is that? Complete the following activity to better understand this type of joint.

INSTRUCTIONS. For each joint type: 1. Identify the joint as _ball-and-socket, condyloid (ellipsoid), gliding, hinge, pivot,_ or _saddle._ 2. Identify the number of planes of movement each type of synovial joint allows as _nonaxial, uniaxial, biaxial,_ or _triaxial._

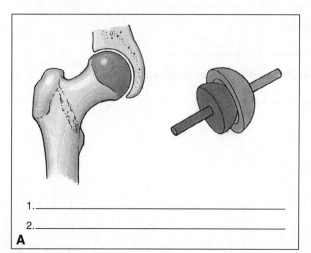

1._____

2._____

A

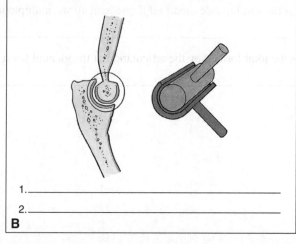

1._____

2._____

B

Figure 2.4

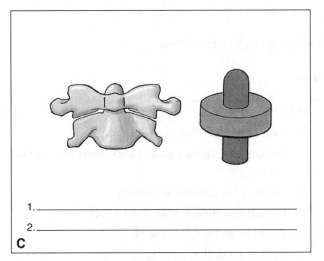

C
1. _____
2. _____

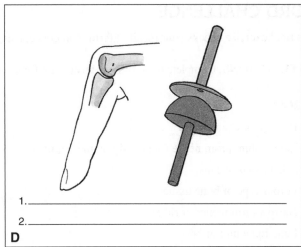

D
1. _____
2. _____

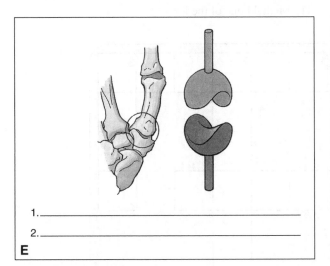

E
1. _____
2. _____

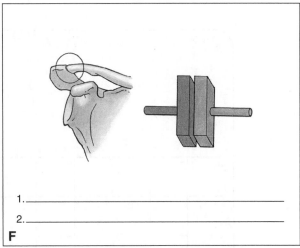

F
1. _____
2. _____

Figure 2.4 (Continued)

DEFINE AND IDENTIFY ACCESSORY MOTIONS

Your study of planes and axes, bones, and joints has helped you understand physiological movements such as flexion and extension. In addition, three accessory motions occur between joint surfaces during physiological movements.

INSTRUCTIONS. Finish the following sentences describing the three benefits of accessory joint motions.

1. They help maintain _____

2. They prevent _____
   between articulating surfaces.

3. They prevent _____
   between articulating surfaces.

INSTRUCTIONS. Label each of the following as an accessory motion or physiological movement by placing the letter A for *accessory* or P for *physiological* in the space provided.

1. _____ Abduction

2. _____ Adduction

3. _____ Depression

4. _____ Elevation

5. _____ Extension

6. _____ External rotation

7. _____ Flexion

8. _____ Glide

9. _____ Internal rotation

10. _____ Pronation

11. _____ Roll

12. _____ Spin

13. _____ Supination

WORD CHALLENGE

This final exercise checks your recall of terms and concepts introduced throughout the chapter.

INSTRUCTIONS. Complete the crossword using the following clues.

ACROSS:

1. Passage or channel.
4. Large, blunt prominence found only on the femur.
7. What *osteo-* means.
8. Porous type of bone tissue.
10. Narrow prominence or ridge.
12. Functional unit of bone.
13. Medial bone of forearm.

DOWN:

2. Type of motion. Roll is an example.
3. Rotation of a surface around a stationary longitudinal axis.
5. One of 24 in the human skeleton.
6. Rounded protrusion from narrow neck.
8. Found between cranial bones.
9. Runs through Haversian canal.
11. Medial bone of the leg.

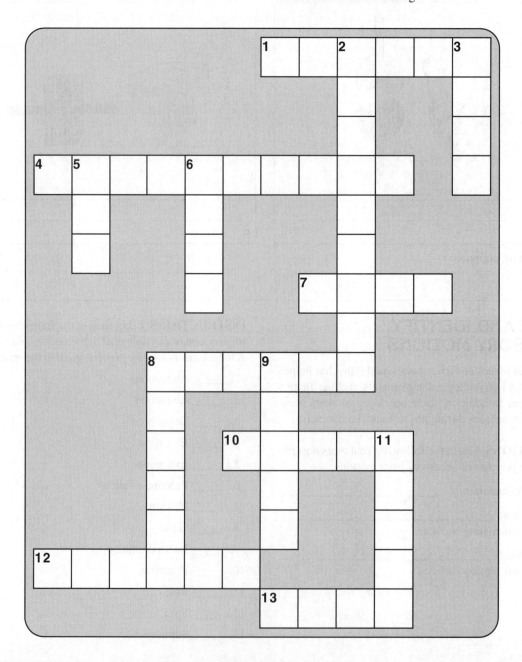

Myology

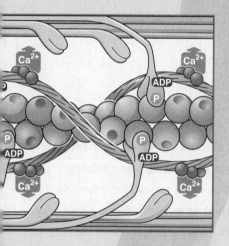

The activities in this chapter will help you study the different types of muscle tissue, their location, and their unique characteristics. You will review skeletal muscle structure, muscle contraction, the different types of contractions, and how individual muscles work together to create movement. Finally, you'll synthesize principles established in Chapters 1 to 3 as you complete activities on levers, proprioception, and range of motion.

COMPARE TYPES OF MUSCLE TISSUE

The following activity will help you compare and contrast the three types of muscle tissue.

INSTRUCTIONS. For each of the three types of muscle tissue, list three characteristics that describe it. Some characteristics may be used more than once.

1. Smooth _____

2. Cardiac _____

3. Skeletal _____

List of Characteristics

Voluntary

Involuntary

Striated

Nonstriated

Short, strong contraction

Moderate, strong contraction

Slow, steady contraction

IDENTIFY SKELETAL MUSCLE FUNCTIONS

You could probably identify one function of skeletal muscle even before you enrolled in this class. This activity should help you remember all five.

INSTRUCTIONS. In the space provided, list the five functions of skeletal muscle. A clue is provided for each function.

1. _____ Clue: This is the one most people know.

2. _____ Clue: Think of leaning over a balcony.

3. _____ Clue: Abdominal muscles have this role.

4. _____ Clue: Think of being outside on a chilly day.

5. _____ Clue: This role helps keep fluids circulating.

IDENTIFY FIBER ARRANGEMENTS

Understanding the way a muscle's fibers are aligned and oriented will help you understand that muscle's function.

INSTRUCTIONS. Label each muscle shown below as *fusiform, circular, triangular, unipennate, bipennate,* or *multipennate.*

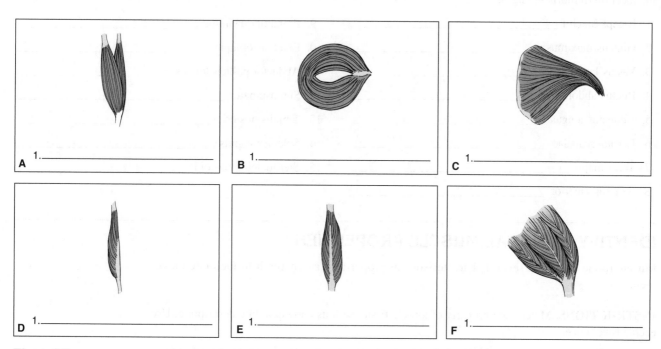

A 1._____

B 1._____

C 1._____

D 1._____

E 1._____

F 1._____

Figure 3.1

INSTRUCTIONS. Match each fiber direction type with its corresponding characteristics. Use each answer one time.

1. _____ Bipennate

2. _____ Circular

3. _____ Fusiform

4. _____ Multipennate

5. _____ Triangular

6. _____ Unipennate

A. Contain several tendons with oblique fibers on both sides that pull from many directions

B. Characterized by a thick central belly and tapered ends that focus force into a specific attachment

C. Fibers start at a broad base and then converge into a specific point, allowing for multiple movements or actions

D. Muscle fibers run at an oblique angle from one side of a central tendon and pull strongly in one direction

E. Fibers surround an opening to form a sphincter, which closes as the muscle contracts and opens when it relaxes.

F. Muscle fibers run at oblique angles on both sides of a central tendon and pull strongly in two directions

PRACTICE NAMING MUSCLES

Muscles are named according to their **f**iber direction, **l**ocation, **a**ction, **s**ize, **s**hape, number of **h**eads, or some combination of these (remember: FLASSH).

INSTRUCTIONS. In the space provided, identify which characteristics are used to name each muscle listed. For example: *rectus femoris* is named for its fiber direction (rectus = straight) and location (femoris = thigh).

1. Biceps brachii _____

2. Gluteus maximus _____

3. Vastus lateralis _____

4. Rectus abdominis _____

5. Adductor longus _____

6. Levator scapulae _____

7. Teres major _____

8. Serratus anterior _____

9. Pronator quadratus _____

10. External oblique _____

11. Abductor pollicis longus _____

12. Supraspinatus _____

13. Tibialis posterior _____

14. Splenius capitis _____

15. Sternocleidomastoid _____

IDENTIFY SKELETAL MUSCLE PROPERTIES

Muscle tissue combines several characteristics or properties that enable it to facilitate movement.

INSTRUCTIONS. Match each property of muscle tissue with its corresponding description. Use each answer once.

1. _____ Conductivity   A. Ability to propagate electrical signals, including action potentials

2. _____ Contractility   B. Ability to respond to a stimulus

3. _____ Elasticity   C. Ability to return to original shape after lengthening or shortening

4. _____ Excitability   D. Ability to shorten or thicken and produce force or movement

5. _____ Extensibility   E. Ability to stretch without sustaining damage

INSTRUCTIONS. In the space provided, draw a picture depicting each of the five properties of muscle tissue: *conductivity, contractility, elasticity, excitability,* and *extensibility.* There is no right answer so be creative! Draw a cartoon or diagram or even the word itself displaying its unique property.

IDENTIFY SKELETAL MUSCLE STRUCTURES

Viewed under a microscope, skeletal muscle tissue reveals several unique structures. Each structure plays an important role in movement.

INSTRUCTIONS. The following diagram depicts muscle tissue both macroscopically and microscopically. Label each of these structures in the correct location on the diagram.

List of Structures

A band
Bone
Endomysium
Epimysium
Fascicle
I band
Mitochondria
Muscle belly
Musculotendinous junction
Myofibril
Nuclei
Nucleus
Perimysium
Sarcolemma (depicted twice)
Sarcoplasm
Sarcoplasmic reticulum
Single muscle fiber
Transverse tubule
Z line

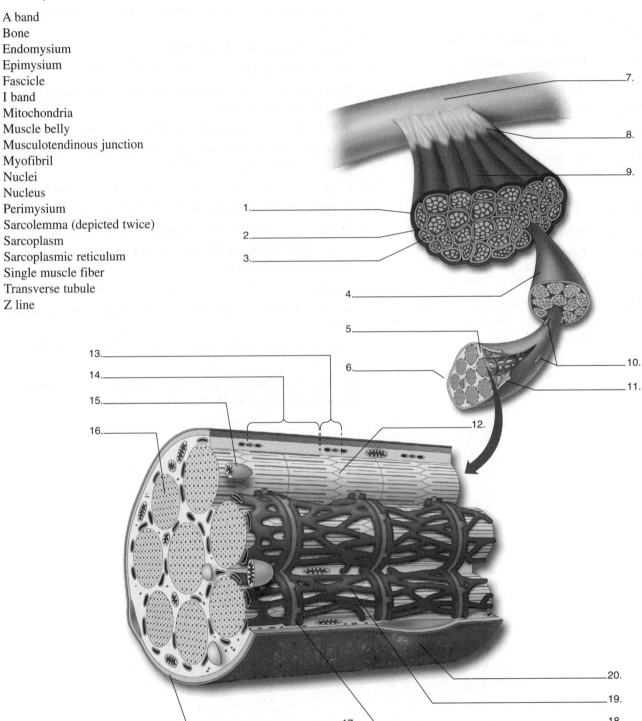

Figure 3.2

INSTRUCTIONS. Match each structure of skeletal muscle tissue with its corresponding function. Use each answer once.

1. _____ Acetylcholine (ACh)

2. _____ Endomysium

3. _____ Epimysium

4. _____ Fascicles

5. _____ Mitochondria

6. _____ Muscle belly

7. _____ Musculotendinous junction

8. _____ Neuromuscular junction

9. _____ Nuclei

10. _____ Perimysium

11. _____ Sarcolemma

12. _____ Sarcomere

13. _____ Sarcoplasm

14. _____ Sarcoplasmic reticulum

15. _____ Synapse

16. _____ Thick filaments

17. _____ Thin filaments

18. _____ Transverse tubules

A. Point where connective tissue surrounding muscle fibers converges and begins forming a tendon

B. Functional unit of a muscle fiber marked by a Z line on each end

C. Transmit nerve impulses from the sarcolemma to the muscle cell interior

D. Connective tissue layer that surrounds fascicles

E. Prevents electrical nerve signals from crossing to the muscle on their own

F. Connects neurons and muscle fibers

G. Connective tissue layer that surrounds entire muscles

H. Neurotransmitter that binds to the sarcolemma and initiates action potential on muscle fibers

I. Stores calcium ions when the muscle fiber is resting

J. Contractile protein containing heads that bind to form cross-bridges and then "pull" to create a power stroke

K. Connective tissue layer that surrounds individual muscle fibers

L. Regulates chemical transport into and out of the cell

M. Produces ATP needed to release energy for muscle contraction

N. Active portion of muscle that lies between tendons and changes shape during contraction

O. Bundles of muscle fibers surrounded by perimysium

P. A gelatinous substance that surrounds the organelles of the muscle cell

Q. Contain the functional information for the cell and control its operations

R. Contractile protein-containing binding sites for cross-bridges and the protein threads that cover them in relaxed muscles

IDENTIFY STRUCTURES AND EVENTS IN MUSCLE CONTRACTION

A series of electrical, chemical, and mechanical interactions occur as the nervous system communicates with the muscular system and a muscle contraction is generated.

INSTRUCTIONS. The following diagrams depict a microscopic view of skeletal muscle proteins at rest (**A**) and during active muscle contraction (**B**). Label each of these structures in the correct location on the diagram.

List of Structures

Actin
Crossbridge
Exposed binding sites
Myosin head
Tropomyosin
Troponin

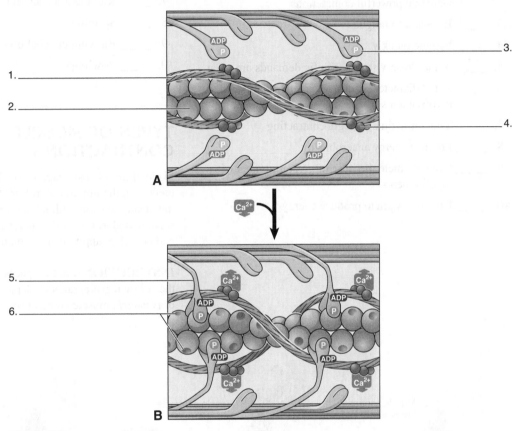

1. _____
2. _____
3. _____
4. _____
5. _____
6. _____

Figure 3.3

INSTRUCTIONS. Place the following events of skeletal muscle contraction in order by numbering them from 1 (occurs first) to 10 (occurs last).

_____ Calcium ions bind to troponin.

_____ Action potential travels down the transverse tubules to the sarcoplasmic reticulum.

_____ Acetylcholine is released from the synaptic vesicles.

_____ Cross-bridges form between actin and myosin.

_____ Action potential travels down the axon of a motor neuron.

_____ Power stroke occurs, pulling the sarcomere together.

_____ Tropomyosin distorts, exposing binding sites on actin.

_____ Acetylcholine molecules bind to receptors on the sarcolemma.

_____ Calcium ions are released from the sarcoplasmic reticulum into the sarcoplasm.

_____ Action potential initiated on muscle cell membrane.

COMPARE SKELETAL MUSCLE FIBER TYPES

The following activities will help you compare and contrast the three types of muscle fibers and their roles in maintaining posture and initiating movement.

INSTRUCTIONS. Match each muscle fiber type with its corresponding properties by placing FT (fast twitch), ST (slow twitch), or IM (intermediate) in the space provided.

1. _____ Metabolically adapt to demands of body

2. _____ Generate powerful contractions

3. _____ Resistant to fatigue

4. _____ Fatigue quickly

5. _____ Act as "reservists" if specific demands are great

6. _____ Small diameter because of smaller number of myofilaments

7. _____ Take more time to begin contracting

8. _____ Produce energy anaerobically

9. _____ Large diameter because of greater number of myofilaments

10. _____ Utilize oxygen to produce energy

INSTRUCTIONS. Identify which type of muscle fiber is used most in each of the following activities by placing FT (fast twitch) or ST (slow twitch) in the space provided.

1. _____ Relaxed walking

2. _____ Folding laundry

3. _____ Whistling a tune

4. _____ Lifting a heavy box

5. _____ Pitching a baseball

6. _____ Standing in line

7. _____ Kicking a soccer ball

8. _____ Sprinting

9. _____ Blowing up a balloon

10. _____ Bowling

TYPES OF MUSCLE CONTRACTIONS

Skeletal muscles are capable of shortening to create movement, lengthening to control or slow movement, and holding steady tension without shortening or lengthening. This section explores the different types of muscle of contraction and how they apply to common movements.

INSTRUCTIONS. In the spaces provided, identify each of the following diagrams as depicting *concentric, eccentric,* or *isometric* muscle contraction.

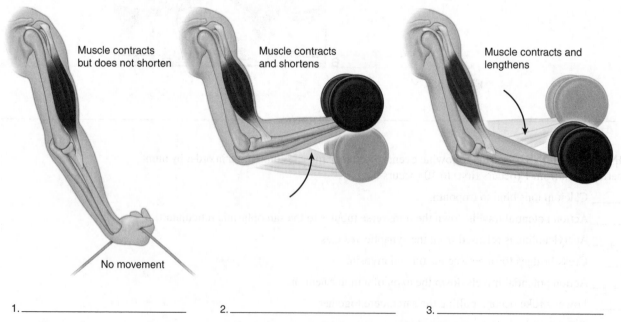

Muscle contracts but does not shorten

Muscle contracts and shortens

Muscle contracts and lengthens

No movement

1. _____   2. _____   3. _____

Figure 3.4

INSTRUCTIONS. In the spaces provided, describe the purpose of each type of muscle contraction.

1. Isometric _____

_____

_____

_____

2. Concentric _____

_____

_____

_____

3. Eccentric _____

_____

_____

_____

Experience Different Types of Muscle Contractions

INSTRUCTIONS. This exercise will help you experience the different types of muscle contractions as they occur in your body. Start by standing up and letting your arms rest at your sides. Place your right hand on the top of your left shoulder so the palm is in contact with your deltoid. Slowly raise your left arm so you are reaching your hand straight out from your shoulder and in front of your body. What is happening to the deltoid as you raise the arm? Try holding your textbook in your left hand as you repeat this exercise to increase the activity of the deltoid and enhance the sensation.

Keep feeling the deltoid as you hold your arm out in front for 30 seconds. Don't move your arm—just keep holding it or the book out in front of you. Is the deltoid working? How? What do you notice about the shape of the muscle? Is there tension? What type of contraction is occurring?

Now, slowly lower your left arm to your side. Can you still feel the deltoid? What happens to the shape and length of the deltoid as you lower your arm? Was this muscle still working as your lowered your arm? What type of contraction allows you to lower your arm to your side? Use the spaces provided to describe what you feel and what type of contraction occurs in each part of this exercise.

1. Raising arm _____

_____

_____

2. Holding arm out _____

_____

_____

3. Lowering arm _____

_____

_____

DEFINE MUSCLE RELATIONSHIPS

Muscles work together to achieve various movements. Understanding the dynamic relationships between muscles helps us better understand complex movement patterns and proper balance between muscles and muscle groups.

INSTRUCTIONS. Use the spaces provided to define the following terms:

1. Agonist _____

_____

_____

2. Synergist _____

_____

_____

3. Antagonist _____

_____

_____

INSTRUCTIONS. Identify opposite actions by placing the letter of one action next to its opposite action.

1. _____ Abduction   A. Adduction

2. _____ Elevation   B. Depression

3. _____ Eversion   C. Dorsiflexion

4. _____ Flexion   D. Extension

5. _____ Medial rotation   E. Inversion

6. _____ Plantarflexion   F. Lateral rotation

7. _____ Pronation   G. Radial deviation

8. _____ Protraction   H. Retraction

9. _____ Ulnar deviation   I. Supination

IDENTIFY MUSCLES OF THE HUMAN BODY

Test your knowledge of muscles in the human body! See how many muscles you can identify from memory. As you label each muscle, practice saying its name correctly, and palpate it if possible.

INSTRUCTIONS. Label the major superficial muscles of the anterior and posterior surface of the body.

Adductors of the thigh	Flexor carpi radialis	Orbicularis oris	Serratus anterior
Biceps brachii	Gastrocnemius	Pectoralis major	Soleus
Brachioradialis	Intercostals	Peroneus longus	Sternocleidomastoid
Deltoid	Internal abdominal oblique	Quadriceps femoris	Temporalis
Extensor carpi radialis	Masseter	Rectus abdominis	Tibialis anterior
External abdominal oblique	Orbicularis oculi	Sartorius	Trapezius

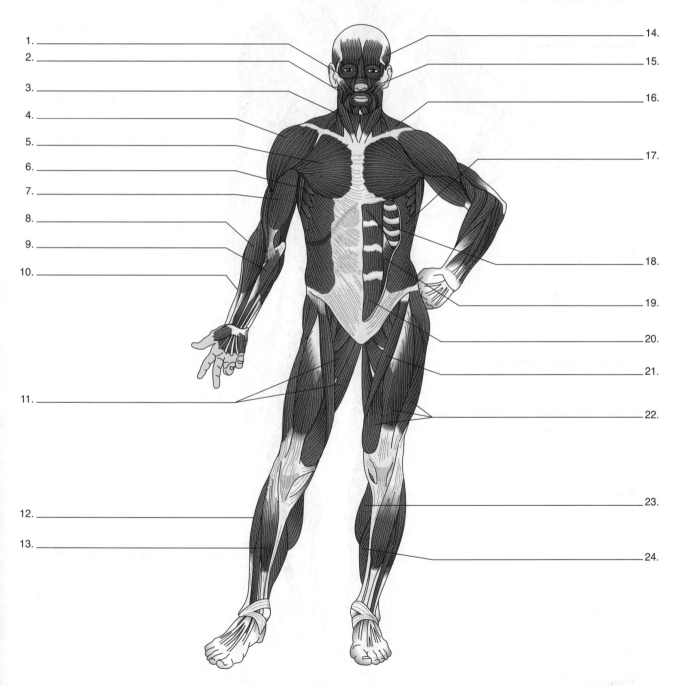

1. _____
2. _____
3. _____
4. _____
5. _____
6. _____
7. _____
8. _____
9. _____
10. _____
11. _____
12. _____
13. _____

14. _____
15. _____
16. _____
17. _____
18. _____
19. _____
20. _____
21. _____
22. _____
23. _____
24. _____

Figure 3.5

Biceps femoris
Deltoid
Gastrocnemius
Gluteus maximus

Gluteus medius
Latissimus dorsi
Peroneus longus
Semimembranosus

Semitendinosus
Sternocleidomastoid
Teres major
Teres minor

Trapezius
Triceps brachii

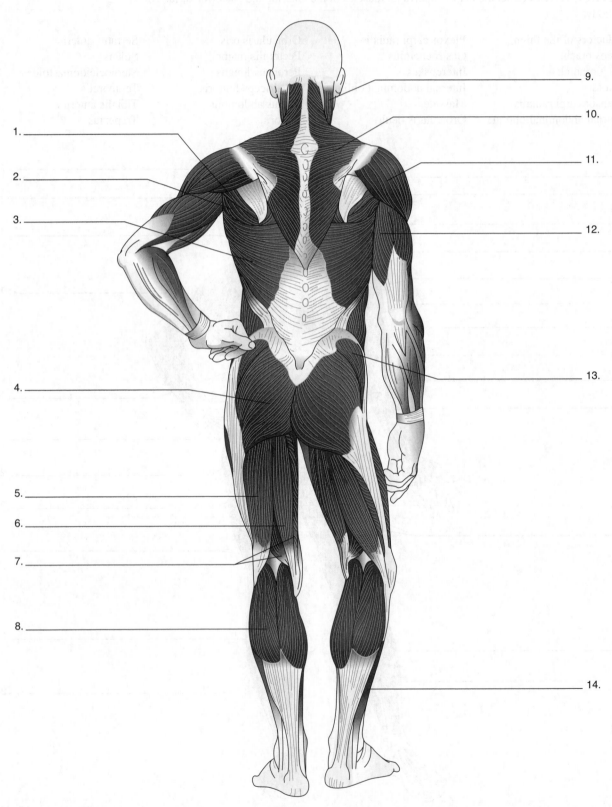

Figure 3.6

CLASSIFY LEVERS

Bones form a rigid system of levers, devices that transmit or modify force to create movement. The following activities explore each part of a lever, how different types of levers function, and how all of this applies to human movement. Let's get started!

INSTRUCTIONS. In the spaces provided, define the following components of a lever. Be sure to identify which anatomic structure in the human body (bones, joints, muscles) acts as each component.

1. Axis/fulcrum: _____

_____

2. Force _____

_____

3. Resistance _____

_____

INSTRUCTIONS. In the spaces provided, draw and label a first-class, second-class, and third-class lever. Be sure and point out the axis, force, and resistance in each of the three drawings.

1. First-class lever

2. Second-class lever

3. Third-class lever

INSTRUCTIONS. List specific examples of first-, second-, and third-class levers in the spaces provided. Include at least one example of each type found in life (e.g., a wrench) and in the body (e.g., the action of biceps brachii on the elbow). Also, describe what quality each type of lever enhances (e.g., speed, range of motion, etc.).

1. First-class lever:

   In life: _____

   _____

   _____

   In the human body: _____

   _____

   _____

   Qualities emphasized: _____

   _____

   _____

2. Second-class lever

   In life: _____

   _____

   _____

   In the human body: _____

   _____

   _____

   Qualities emphasized: _____

   _____

   _____

3. Third-class lever

   In life: _____

   _____

   _____

   In the human body: _____

   _____

   _____

   Qualities emphasized: _____

   _____

   _____

CLASSIFY PROPRIOCEPTORS

Skeletal muscles provide force to move levers in the human body, but they do not work alone. The following activities examine how the nervous system monitors and controls the posture, positioning, and movement of these levers.

INSTRUCTIONS. Pair each of the following proprioceptors with the corresponding location in the human body. Use each answer one time.

1. _____ Golgi tendon organ

2. _____ Muscle spindle

3. _____ Pacinian corpuscle

4. _____ Ruffini ending

5. _____ Vestibular apparatus

A. Inner ear

B. Skeletal muscle fibers

C. Joint capsules

D. Skin, connective tissue, muscles, tendons

E. Connective tissue of tendons

INSTRUCTIONS. Re-organize the following table to correctly pair the proprioceptors with the corresponding stimulus or trigger and the resulting response to that trigger. Use each answer one time.

Structure	Stimulus or Trigger	Response to Trigger
Golgi tendon organ	Vibration and deep pressure	Indicates position of joint
Muscle spindle	Change in head position	Contracts muscle
Pacinian corpuscle	Rapid change in muscle length	Inhibits muscle contraction
Ruffini ending	Distortion of joint capsule	Reestablishes equilibrium
Vestibular apparatus	Excessive muscle contraction	Indicates direction and speed of movement

Structure	Stimulus or Trigger	Response to Trigger
Golgi tendon organ		
Muscle spindle		
Pacinian corpuscle		
Ruffini ending		
Vestibular apparatus		

RANGE OF MOTION

Let's wrap up our introduction to anatomy, physiology, and kinesiology by exploring range of motion (ROM). The following activities help deepen your understanding of joint movement and evaluating the health and function of surrounding structures.

INSTRUCTIONS. First, let's take a look at **why** we perform or have clients perform various movements as an integral part of bodywork. This is clarified when you understand what you are looking for as you perform each type of ROM assessment. In the spaces provided, describe the purpose of each type of ROM.

1. Active range of motion (AROM)

   _____

   _____

2. Passive range of motion (PROM)

   _____

   _____

3. Resisted range of motion (RROM)

   _____

   _____

INSTRUCTIONS. In the spaces provided, describe what the client should be doing during the ROM assessment. Next, describe what you, the practitioner, should be doing.

1. Active range of motion (AROM):

   Client: _____

   _____

   Practitioner: _____

   _____

2. Passive range of motion (PROM):

   Client: _____

   _____

   Practitioner: _____

   _____

3. Resisted range of motion (RROM):

   Client: _____

   _____

   Practitioner: _____

   _____

WORD CHALLENGE

This final exercise checks your recall of terms and concepts introduced throughout the chapter.

INSTRUCTIONS. Fifteen terms introduced in this chapter are hidden in the word search puzzle. Locate each term and write it next to its numbered definition. Terms may be found horizontally, vertically, or diagonally.

List of Terms

1. Overall awareness of body position _____
   _____

2. Muscle most responsible for creating a movement (also called *prime mover*) _____
   _____

3. Motor neuron and all the fibers it controls _____
   _____

4. Network of channels that store calcium ions _____
   _____

5. Ability to stretch without sustaining damage _____
   _____

6. Feather-shaped _____
   _____

7. Gap between axon branches and muscle fibers _____
   _____

8. Type of skeletal muscle fiber that produces fast, powerful contractions but quickly fatigues _____
   _____

9. Muscle contractions that generate tension in a muscle but does not create joint movement _____
   _____

10. A wheelbarrow is a common example _____
    _____

11. Location of vestibular apparatus _____
    _____

12. Perceived quality of movement at the end of a joint's available range of motion _____
    _____

13. Type of energy production that uses oxygen _____
    _____

14. Globular protein essential for muscle contraction ____
    _____

15. Bundle of muscle fibers _____
    _____

```
R B N G Y L C R N G O D I P P D W R X - X H
Y T G G I X S N O I T P E C O I R P O R P H
T R Y M B H G M T W T V F A S C I C L E V C
U C I R T E M O S I N G R E N N D Y - A I T
I A E O X X D C T O E N V A X M G H H Y N I
A X I X P E G - I I V S O Y M - M W G P G W
O S F B E T A L C N N B C I H U U A G M C T
W G F N S C L Y - N N U I R E N D F E E L T
E L Y B P V V C S U W E R P X I S R R A I S
M N I E A W - X H O N A R O E M U W G F G A
W V E N N O P H H S Y R I E T R U V E B W F
T G W T Y E O P P W G U T V A O I M Y H G I
I M T F S - M Y H B I R G R L R M P W U O O
M U L U C I T E R C I M S A L P O C R A S V
V G B M D F N G B B W R I F D F M L X G S T
E N H P M M A L B Y L - F L I B E C H F I V
V B S H T A L X I S M E W Y V E N F W B M N
V W A S V V B W O E A Y E Y B L - F U H S I
A U I A U V M X T C P - O I B Y V T G Y C X
L R E C F N D A I Y F F N A O F F S E H C C
I F X T I X N E T R N T B F G T H F X V I S
T C B I F N Y D W O S C T C P O V R F O B W
L I X N E R M V P O H N T S L M N M D R O F
F X H P W V - B A Y T T W U O N E I O M R W
C - V X A P C P R M Y L R F G S H S S O E E
S G Y E Y T I L I B I S N E T X E P D T A V
S R B C W Y O U E R M L U - B P Y M P R V -
R F T O S E C O N D - C L A S S L E V E R O
```

Shoulder

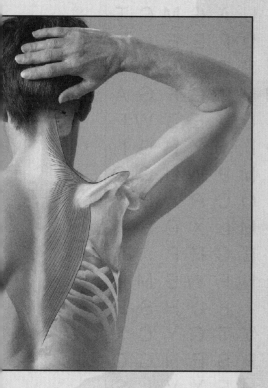

The shoulder is a complex structure composed of several joints, capable of multiple actions, and requiring coordinated efforts of various muscles. When functioning properly, the shoulder seamlessly shifts between stability and mobility. The following activities will help you appreciate the structure and function of the shoulder.

4

LABEL SURFACE LANDMARKS

This activity will assist you in orienting yourself during palpation and visually assessing the health and function of underlying structures.

INSTRUCTIONS. The following images depict the major surface landmarks in the shoulder region. Label each of the following in the spaces provided.

List of Structures, Anterior View

Axilla
Biceps brachii
Clavicle
Pectoralis major
Serratus anterior
Sternum

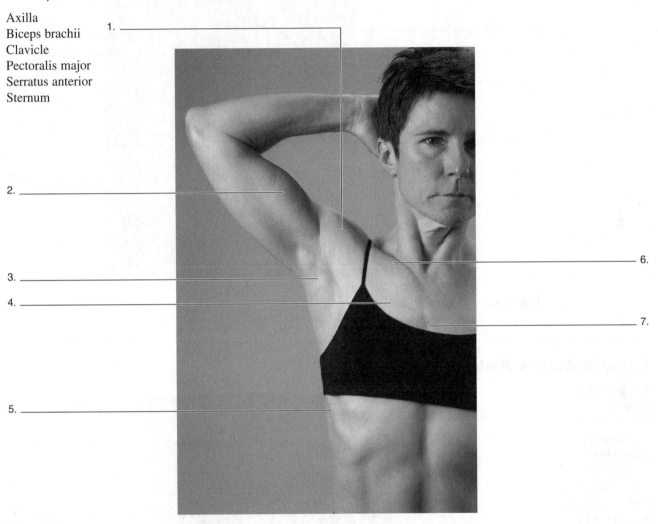

1. _____

2. _____

3. _____

4. _____

5. _____

6. _____

7. _____

Figure 4.1

List of Structures, Lateral View

Acromion
  process
Biceps brachii
Clavicle
Deltoid
Sternum
Triceps brachii

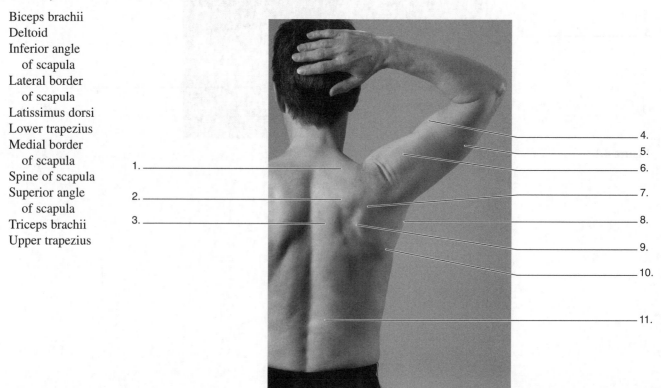

1. _____

2. _____

3. _____

4. _____

5. _____

6. _____

Figure 4.2

List of Structures, Posterior View

Biceps brachii
Deltoid
Inferior angle
  of scapula
Lateral border
  of scapula
Latissimus dorsi
Lower trapezius
Medial border
  of scapula
Spine of scapula
Superior angle
  of scapula
Triceps brachii
Upper trapezius

1. _____

2. _____

3. _____

4. _____

5. _____

6. _____

7. _____

8. _____

9. _____

10. _____

11. _____

Figure 4.3

COLOR AND LABEL SKELETAL STRUCTURES

Bones and bony landmarks provide consistent touchstones as we locate, differentiate, and explore soft-tissue structures such as muscles, tendons, and ligaments.

INSTRUCTIONS. Color and label each of the following bones and bony landmarks for the shoulder region.

List of Structures, Anterior View

Acromioclavicular joint
Acromion process
Clavicle
Coracoid process
Costocartilage
Glenohumeral joint
Head of the humerus
Manubrium of sternum
Scapula
Sternoclavicular joint
Sternum

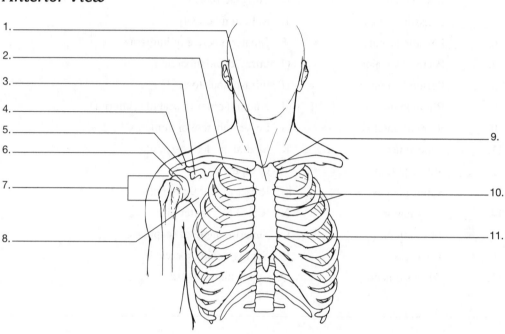

Figure 4.4

List of Structures, Posterior View

Acromion process
Clavicle
Head of humerus
Infraspinous fossa
Shaft of humerus
Spine of scapula
Supraspinous fossa

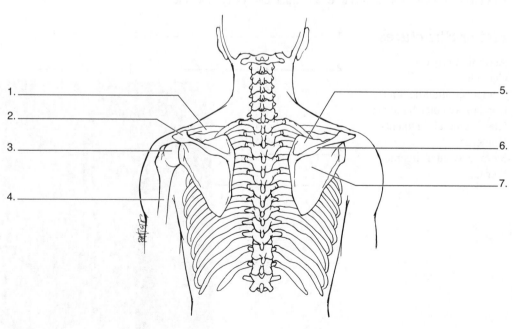

Figure 4.5

MATCH MUSCLES AND BONY LANDMARKS

INSTRUCTIONS. Match each of the following bony landmarks with the corresponding muscle attachment. Use each answer one time.

1. _____ Biceps brachii
2. _____ Coracobrachialis
3. _____ Deltoid
4. _____ Infraspinatus
5. _____ Latissimus dorsi
6. _____ Levator scapula
7. _____ Pectoralis major
8. _____ Pectoralis minor
9. _____ Rhomboids
10. _____ Serratus anterior
11. _____ Subclavius
12. _____ Subscapularis
13. _____ Supraspinatus
14. _____ Teres major
15. _____ Teres minor
16. _____ Trapezius
17. _____ Triceps brachii

A. Bicipital groove (lateral lip)
B. Bicipital groove (medial lip)
C. Clavicle (inferior surface)
D. Coracoid process
E. Deltoid tuberosity
F. Greater tubercle of humerus
G. Infraglenoid tubercle
H. Infraspinous fossa
I. Lateral border of scapula (inferior)
J. Lesser tubercle of humerus
K. Medial border of scapula
L. Occiput
M. Ribs 1 to 8 or 9 (lateral)
N. Ribs 3 to 5 (anterior)
O. Superior angle of scapula
P. Supraglenoid tubercle
Q. Supraspinous fossa

LABEL JOINTS AND LIGAMENTS

This next activity will help you explore the joints of the shoulder regions and the ligaments that hold them together.

INSTRUCTIONS. Label the bones and ligaments of the shoulder:

List of Structures

Acromion process
Clavicle
Coracoacromial ligament
Coracoclavicular ligaments
Glenohumeral ligaments
Humerus
Sternoclavicular ligament
Sternum

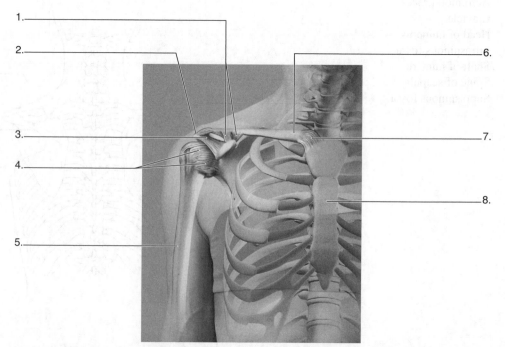

Figure 4.6

COMPLETE THE TABLE: LIGAMENTS

Fill in the missing information about ligaments of the shoulder. The first column indicates a ligament of the shoulder, the second identifies which bony landmarks it joins, and the third indicates the function of the ligament or what movements are limited by this structure. The first row is completed for you as an example.

Ligament	Bony Landmarks Joined	Function
Acromioclavicular	Lateral clavicle Acromion process	Anchors lateral clavicle to scapula, preventing elevation of lateral clavicle
Coracoacromial		
Coracoclavicular		
Coracohumeral		
Glenohumeral		
Sternoclavicular		

LABEL MUSCLES OF THE SHOULDER

Both the anterior and posterior shoulder are superficially covered by large, multifunctional muscles. These broad muscles anchor the shoulder girdle to the neck and chest, power movements in multiple directions, and fix or glide the scapula as the arm moves. Deeper muscles steer the humerus or further fix the scapula as the superficial muscles power movement.

INSTRUCTIONS. The following diagrams depict the superficial muscles of the shoulder. Label each of the following structures.

List of Structures, Anterior View

Biceps brachii
Coracobrachialis
Deltoid
Pectoralis major
Serratus anterior
Trapezius

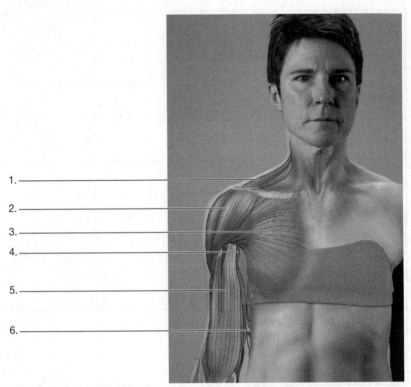

Figure 4.7

List of Structures, Posterior View

Deltoid
Infraspinatus
Latissimus dorsi
Teres major
Teres minor
Trapezius
Triceps brachii
    (lateral head)
Triceps brachii
    (long head)
Triceps brachii
    (medial head)

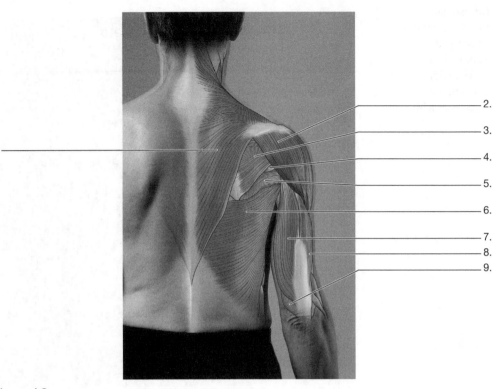

Figure 4.8

INSTRUCTIONS. The following diagrams depict the deep muscles of the shoulder. Label each of the following structures.

List of Structures, Anterior View

Biceps brachii
Coracobrachialis
Pectoralis minor
Serratus anterior
Subclavius
Subscapularis
Teres major
Teres minor

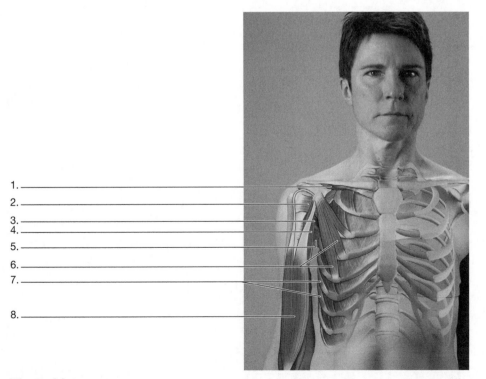

Figure 4.9

List of Structures, Posterior View

Infraspinatus
Levator scapula
Rhomboid
Supraspinatus
Teres major
Teres minor
Triceps brachii

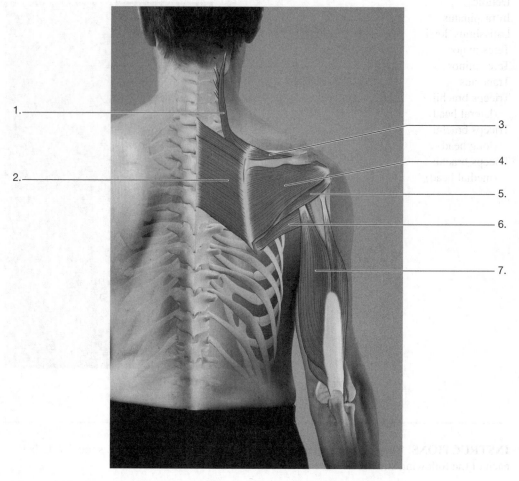

1.

2.

3.

4.

5.

6.

7.

Figure 4.10

LABEL SPECIAL STRUCTURES

This exercise will help you become aware of blood vessels, lymph nodes and vessels, and nerves as well as mammary tissue in the shoulder area.

INSTRUCTIONS. Label each of the following special structures in the shoulder region.

List of Structures

Axillary lymph nodes
Brachial artery
Brachial vein
Clavicle
Common carotid artery

Deep cervical lymph nodes
Internal jugular vein
Mammary tissue
Parasternal lymph nodes
Pectoralis major

Pectoralis minor
Serratus anterior
Subclavian artery and vein
Supraclavicular lymph nodes

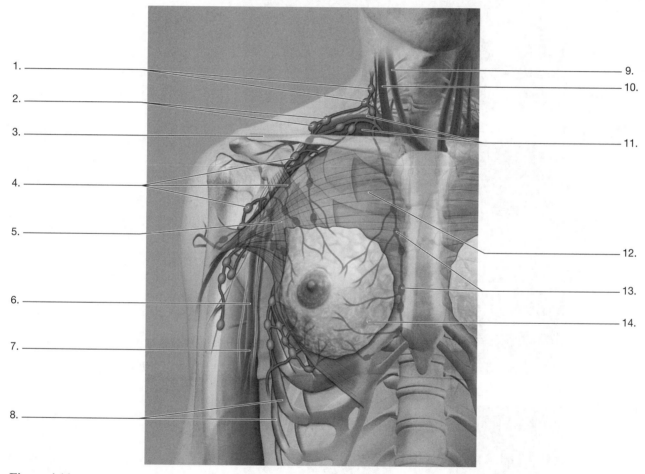

1. _____
2. _____
3. _____
4. _____
5. _____
6. _____
7. _____
8. _____

9. _____
10. _____
11. _____
12. _____
13. _____
14. _____

Figure 4.11

IDENTIFY SHOULDER MOVEMENTS

The scapulothoracic joint and the glenohumeral joint work together to produce the large, sweeping movements of the shoulder.

INSTRUCTIONS. Beneath each of the following figures, write the name of each motion.

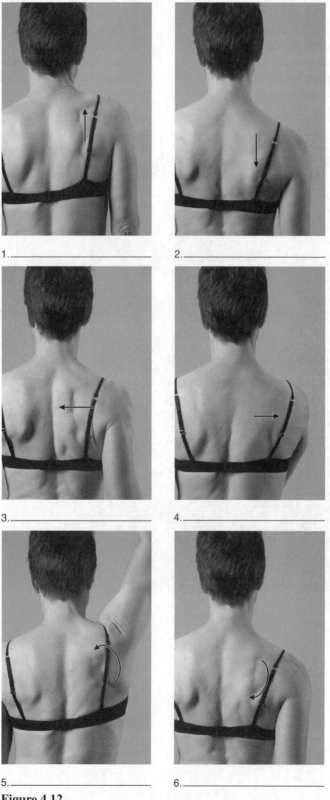

1._____ 2._____

3._____ 4._____

5._____ 6._____

Figure 4.12

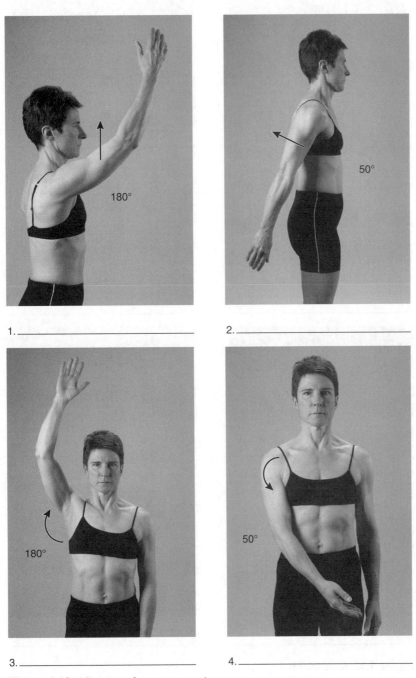

1. _____

2. _____

3. _____

4. _____

Figure 4.13 (*Continued on next page*)

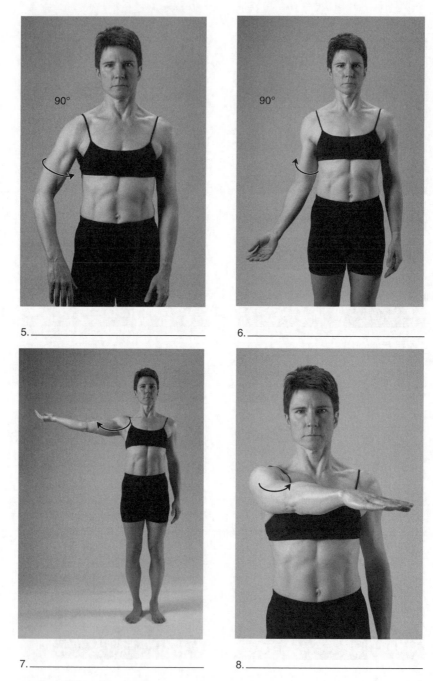

5. _____   6. _____

7. _____   8. _____

Figure 4.13 (*continued*)

MATCH MUSCLE ORIGINS, INSERTIONS, AND ACTIONS

Each muscle has unique muscle attachments, crosses a specific joint or joints, and performs specific movements.

INSTRUCTIONS. Match each shoulder muscle with the corresponding origin. Use each answer one time.

1. _____ Biceps brachii
2. _____ Coracobrachialis
3. _____ Deltoid
4. _____ Infraspinatus
5. _____ Latissimus dorsi
6. _____ Levator scapulae
7. _____ Pectoralis major
8. _____ Pectoralis minor
9. _____ Rhomboids
10. _____ Serratus anterior
11. _____ Subclavius
12. _____ Subscapularis
13. _____ Supraspinatus
14. _____ Teres major
15. _____ Teres minor
16. _____ Trapezius
17. _____ Triceps brachii

A. First rib at junction with costocartilage
B. Coracoid process of scapula
C. Inferior lateral border of scapula
D. Infraglenoid tubercle of scapula and posterior shaft of humerus
E. Infraspinous fossa of scapula
F. Lateral one-third of clavicle, acromion process, spine of the scapula
G. Medial clavicle, sternum, costocartilages of ribs 1–7
H. Occiput, nuchal ligament, spinous processes of C7–T12
I. Outer surfaces of upper 8 or 9 ribs
J. Ribs 3–5
K. Spinous processes of C7–T5
L. Spinous processes T7–L5, posterior iliac crest, posterior sacrum
M. Subscapular fossa
N. Superior lateral border of scapula
O. Supraglenoid tubercle and coracoid process of scapula
P. Supraspinous fossa of scapula
Q. Transverse processes of C1–4

INSTRUCTIONS. Match each shoulder muscle with the corresponding insertion. Some answers will be used more than once.

1. _____ Biceps brachii
2. _____ Coracobrachialis
3. _____ Deltoid
4. _____ Infraspinatus
5. _____ Latissimus dorsi
6. _____ Levator scapulae
7. _____ Pectoralis major
8. _____ Pectoralis minor
9. _____ Rhomboids
10. _____ Serratus anterior
11. _____ Subclavius
12. _____ Subscapularis
13. _____ Supraspinatus
14. _____ Teres major
15. _____ Teres minor
16. _____ Trapezius
17. _____ Triceps brachii

A. Coracoid process of scapula
B. Deltoid tuberosity
C. Greater tubercle of humerus (use this answer three times)
D. Lateral one-third of clavicle, acromion process, spine of scapula
E. Lateral lip of bicipital groove
F. Lesser tubercle of humerus
G. Medial border of scapula (costal surface)
H. Medial border of scapula (root of spine to inferior angle)
I. Medial lip of bicipital groove (use this answer twice)
J. Middle one-third of inferior clavicle
K. Middle one-third of medial shaft of humerus
L. Olecranon process of ulna
M. Radial tuberosity and bicipital aponeurosis
N. Superior angle of scapula

INSTRUCTIONS. Match each shoulder muscle with the corresponding actions. Choose all that apply. Some answers will be used more than once.

1. _____ Biceps brachii
2. _____ Coracobrachialis
3. _____ Deltoid
4. _____ Infraspinatus
5. _____ Latissimus dorsi
6. _____ Levator scapulae
7. _____ Pectoralis major
8. _____ Pectoralis minor
9. _____ Rhomboids
10. _____ Serratus anterior
11. _____ Subclavius
12. _____ Subscapularis
13. _____ Supraspinatus
14. _____ Teres major
15. _____ Teres minor
16. _____ Trapezius
17. _____ Triceps brachii

A. Extends the head and neck
B. Laterally flexes the head and neck
C. Rotates the head and neck to opposite side
D. Rotates the head and neck to same side
E. Scapular depression
F. Scapular downward rotation
G. Scapular elevation
H. Scapular protraction
I. Scapular retraction
J. Scapular upward rotation
K. Shoulder abduction
L. Shoulder adduction
M. Shoulder extension
N. Shoulder external rotation
O. Shoulder flexion
P. Shoulder horizontal abduction
Q. Shoulder horizontal adduction
R. Shoulder internal rotation

IDENTIFY SHORTENING AND LENGTHENING SHOULDER MUSCLES

This activity will help you become more familiar with each muscle of the shoulder.

INSTRUCTIONS. For each of the following muscles, identify the position where the muscle is most shortened and the position that lengthens or stretches the muscle. The first one is completed as an example.

Biceps Brachii

Shortened position = shoulder and elbow flexed and forearm supinated
Lengthened position = shoulder and elbow extended and forearm pronated

Latissimus Dorsi

Shortened position = _____

_____

Lengthened position = _____

_____

Pectoralis Major

Shortened position = _____

_____

Lengthened position = _____

_____

Pectoralis Minor

Shortened position = _____

_____

Lengthened position = _____

_____

Rhomboids

Shortened position = _____

_____

Lengthened position = _____

_____

Subscapularis

Shortened position = _____

_____

Lengthened position = _____

_____

Supraspinatus

Shortened position = _____

_____

Lengthened position = _____

_____

Teres Major

Shortened position = _____

_____

Lengthened position = _____

_____

Triceps Brachii

Shortened position = _____

_____

Lengthened position = _____

_____

COMPLETE THE TABLE: SYNERGISTS/ANTAGONISTS

Recall that synergist muscles work together. Antagonists work in opposition.

INSTRUCTIONS. Fill in the missing information about muscles of the shoulder. The first column indicates a movement of the shoulder, the second identifies which muscles perform this action, and the third indicates the opposite action. The first row is completed for you as an example.

Movement	Muscles	Opposite Action
Scapular depression	Trapezius (lower fibers) Pectoralis minor Serratus anterior	Scapular elevation
Scapular downward rotation		
Scapular elevation		
Scapular protraction		
Scapular retraction		

(*Continued on next page*)

Movement	Muscles	Opposite Action
Scapular upward rotation		
Shoulder abduction		
Shoulder adduction		
Shoulder extension		
Shoulder external rotation		
Shoulder flexion		
Shoulder horizontal abduction		
Shoulder horizontal adduction		
Shoulder internal rotation		

PUTTING THE SHOULDER IN MOTION

The following activity brings together all that you have learned about the shoulder. For each movement, describe the joints involved, the joint motions that occur, and the sequence in which they occur. It is often helpful to perform the movement yourself, observe someone else performing the movement, or watch an animation or video of the movement to better understand what is happening and when. The following example is completed for you.

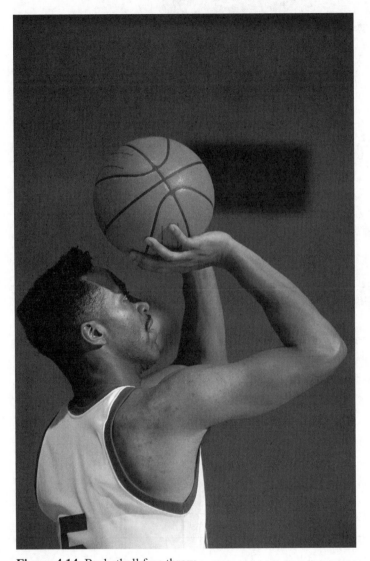

Figure 4.14 Basketball free throw

INSTRUCTIONS. List the joints involved in the movement shown:

Shoulder	Hips
Elbow	Knees
Wrist	Ankles

INSTRUCTIONS. List the motions that occur at each joint.

Shoulder flexion	Hips extension
Elbow extension	Knees extension
Wrist flexion	Ankles plantarflexion

INSTRUCTIONS. List the sequence of events that make up this movement:

1. The hips and the knees extend as the ankles plantarflex, "lifting" the entire upper body.

2. The shoulder flexes until the elbow is even with the face and the ball is level with the forehead.

3. The elbow and the wrist extend to push the ball up and forward toward the basket until the ball rolls off the fingertips.

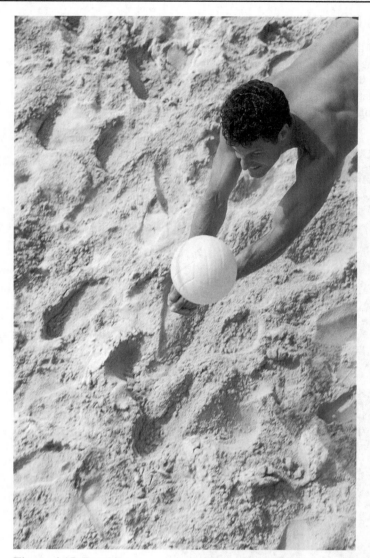

Figure 4.15 Reaching

INSTRUCTIONS. List the joints involved in the movement shown:

_____

_____

_____

INSTRUCTIONS. List the motions that occur at each joint:

_____

_____

_____

INSTRUCTIONS. List the sequence of events that make up this movement:

_____

_____

_____

_____

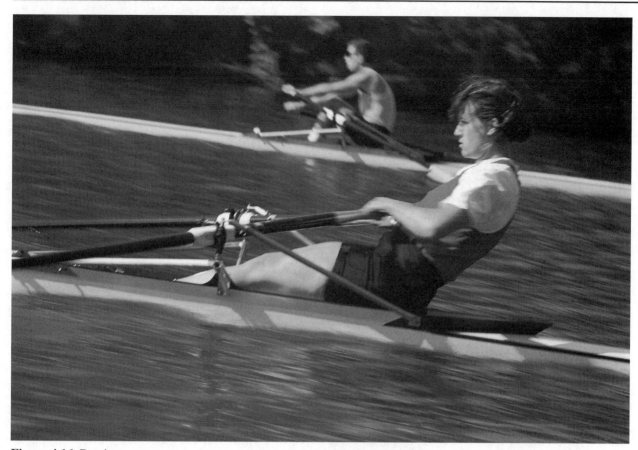

Figure 4.16 Rowing

INSTRUCTIONS. List the joints involved in the movement shown:

_____

_____

_____

INSTRUCTIONS. List the motions that occur at each joint:

_____

_____

_____

INSTRUCTIONS. List the sequence of events that make up this movement:

_____

_____

_____

_____

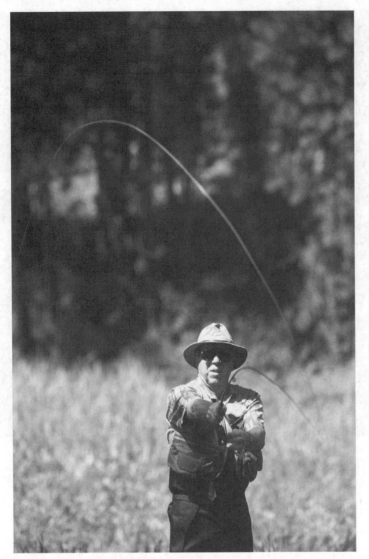

Figure 4.17 Casting a line

INSTRUCTIONS. List the joints involved in the movement shown:

_____

_____

_____

INSTRUCTIONS. List the motions that occur at each joint:

_____

_____

_____

INSTRUCTIONS. List the sequence of events that make up this movement:

_____

_____

_____

_____

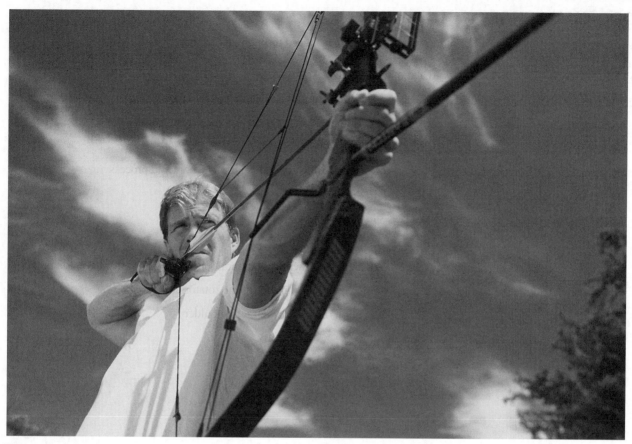

Figure 4.18 Drawing a bow

INSTRUCTIONS. List the joints involved in the movement shown:

_____

_____

_____

INSTRUCTIONS. List the motions that occur at each joint:

_____

_____

_____

INSTRUCTIONS. List the sequence of events that make up this movement:

_____

_____

_____

_____

WORD CHALLENGE

This final exercise checks your recall of terms and concepts introduced throughout the chapter.

INSTRUCTIONS. Unscramble each word and match it to its description.

1. usumerh _____   A. Bundle of nerve fibers in the shoulder

2. nabmumuri _____   B. Prime mover for nearly all movements of the shoulder

3. steer nroim _____   C. Insertion of deltoid

4. alcaups _____   D. Tethers the humeral head to the coracoid process

5. subarcoilma subar _____   E. Armpit

6. didetol _____   F. Most superior portion of the sternum

7. stiazepru _____   G. Shoulder blade

8. lalaix _____   H. Separates the glenohumeral joint capsule and the acromion process

9. ruomhacercoal gainmelt _____   I. One of four muscles of the rotator cuff

10. crabalih lsxupe _____   J. With rhomboids, retracts shoulder

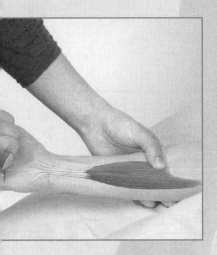

Elbow, Forearm, Wrist, and Hand

5

It is time to travel distally, away from the shoulder, down the upper extremity and toward the hand. Whereas the shoulder is designed for maximal range of motion and positional versatility, elbow and forearm hinging and pivoting transfer force along a single plane, strongly directing efforts in one direction. As joints and muscles become smaller in the wrist and hand, more subtle motions are possible. The activities in this chapter will help you appreciate the structure and function of the elbow, forearm, wrist, and hand.

LABEL SURFACE LANDMARKS

This activity will assist you in orienting yourself during palpation and visually assessing the health and function of underlying structures.

INSTRUCTIONS. The following images depict the major surface landmarks of the arm. Label each of the following in the spaces provided.

List of Structures, Anterior View

Brachialis
Brachioradialis
Cubital fossa
Flexor carpi radialis
Flexor carpi ulnaris
Flexor tendons
Medial epicondyle
Olecranon process
Palmaris longus
Pisiform
Radial styloid
    process

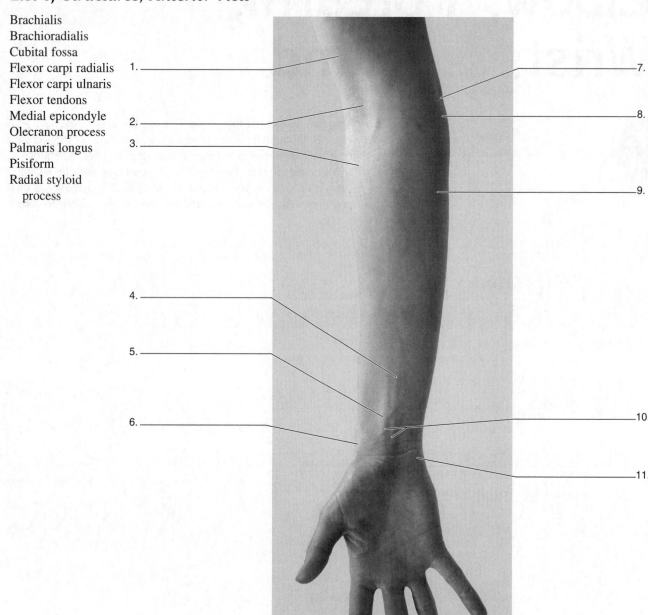

1. _____
2. _____
3. _____
4. _____
5. _____
6. _____

7. _____
8. _____
9. _____
10. _____
11. _____

Figure 5.1

List of Structures, Posterior View

Anconeus
Brachioradialis
Extensor carpi
   radialis longus
   and brevis
Extensor carpi ulnaris
Extensor digitorum
Lateral epicondyle
Olecranon process
Radial styloid process
Ulnar styloid process

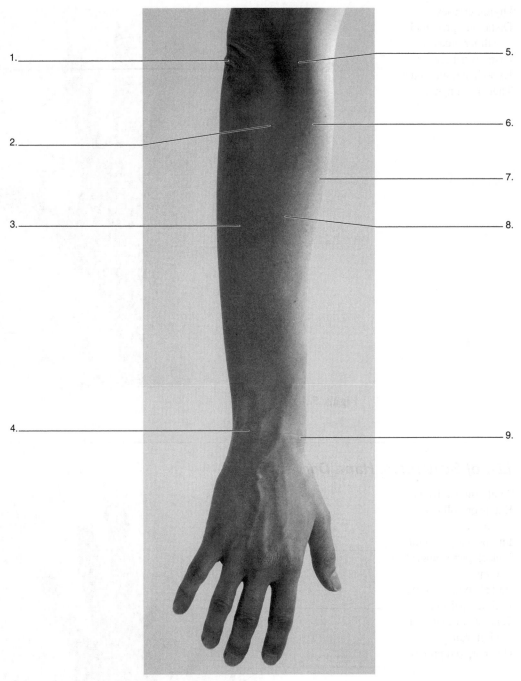

Figure 5.2

List of Structures, Hand Palmar View

Digital creases
Distal and proximal
    palmar creases
Distal wrist crease
Hypothenar eminence
Thenar eminence

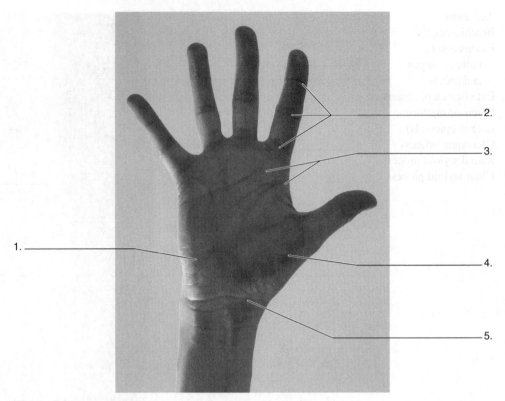

Figure 5.3

List of Structures, Hand Dorsal View

Anatomic snuffbox
Extensor pollicis
    longus
Interphalangeal joints
Metacarpophalangeal
    joints
Radial styloid process
Radiocarpal joint
Tendons of extensor
    digitorum
Ulnar styloid process

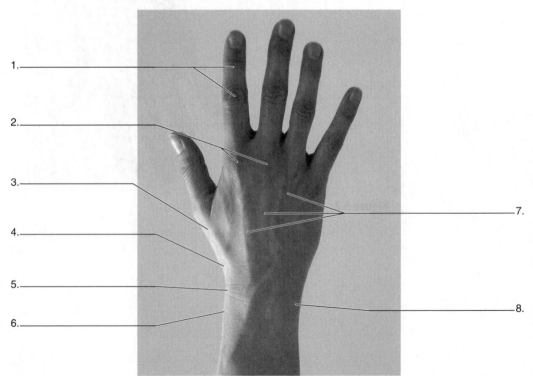

Figure 5.4

IDENTIFY SKELETAL STRUCTURES

The following exercises will help you identify structures below the surface. Bones and bony landmarks provide consistent touchstones for exploration of soft-tissue structures such as muscles, tendons, and ligaments.

INSTRUCTIONS. The following images depict the bones and bony landmarks for the elbow, forearm, wrist, and hand. Color and label each of the following structures.

List of Structures, Forearm Anterior View

Carpals	Medial epicondyle	Radial tuberosity
Coronoid process	Metacarpals	Radiocarpal joint
Humerus	Phalanges	Radius
Lateral epicondyle	Radial head	Ulna

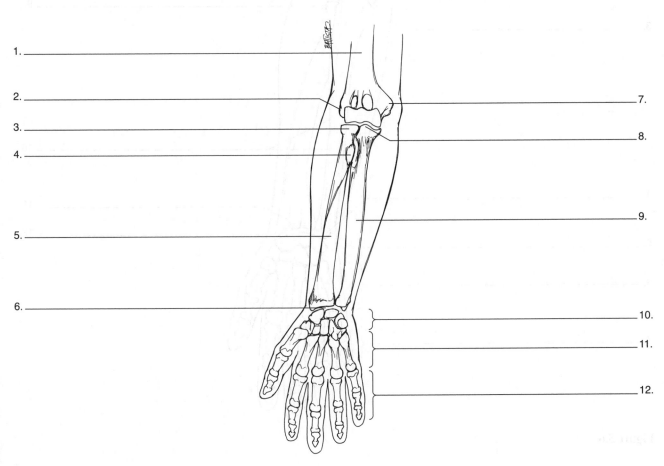

1. _____

2. _____

3. _____

4. _____

5. _____

6. _____

7. _____

8. _____

9. _____

10. _____

11. _____

12. _____

Figure 5.5

List of Structures, Forearm Posterior View

Carpals
Lateral epicondyle
Lister tubercle
Medial epicondyle

Metacarpals
Olecranon fossa
Olecranon process of ulna
Phalanges

Radial head
Radial styloid process
Ulnar ridge
Ulnar styloid process

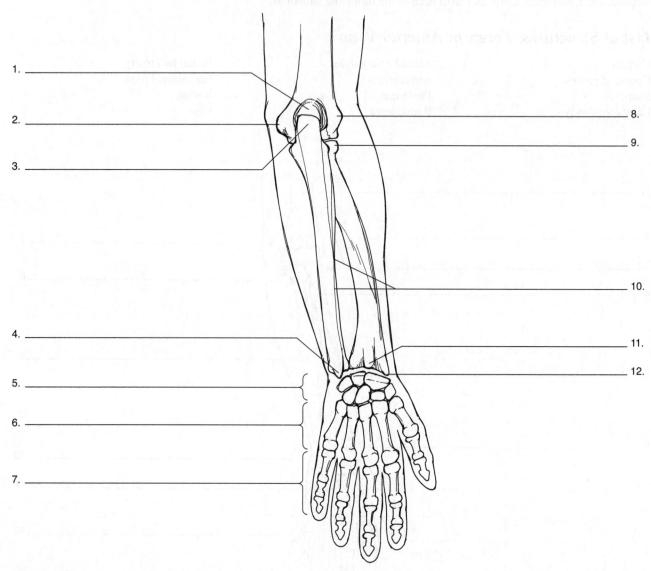

1. _____
2. _____
3. _____
4. _____
5. _____
6. _____
7. _____

8. _____
9. _____
10. _____
11. _____
12. _____

Figure 5.6

List of Structures, Hand Palmar View

Capitate
First distal phalange
First metacarpal
First proximal phalange
Fifth distal phalange
Fifth metacarpal
Fifth middle phalange

Fifth proximal phalange
Hamate
Lunate
Pisiform
Radial styloid process
Radius
Scaphoid

Trapezium
Trapezoid
Triquetrum
Ulna
Ulnar styloid process

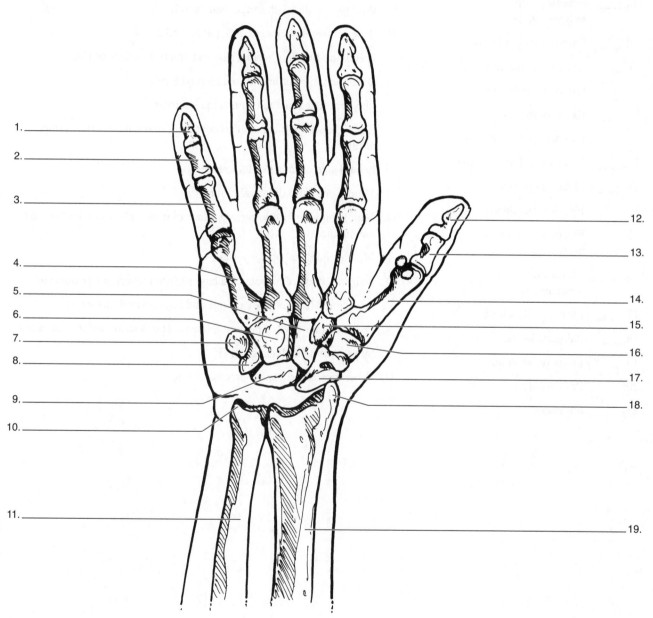

1.
2.
3.
4.
5.
6.
7.
8.
9.
10.
11.

12.
13.
14.
15.
16.
17.
18.
19.

Figure 5.7

INSTRUCTIONS. Match each of the following bony landmarks with the corresponding muscle attachment. Use each answer one time.

1. _____ Abductor pollicis longus

2. _____ Anconeus

3. _____ Brachialis

4. _____ Brachioradialis

5. _____ Extensor carpi radialis brevis

6. _____ Extensor carpi radialis longus

7. _____ Extensor carpi ulnaris

8. _____ Extensor digiti minimi

9. _____ Extensor digitorum

10. _____ Extensor indicis

11. _____ Extensor pollicis brevis

12. _____ Extensor pollicis longus

13. _____ Flexor carpi radialis

14. _____ Flexor carpi ulnaris

15. _____ Flexor digitorum profundus

16. _____ Flexor digitorum superficialis

17. _____ Flexor pollicis longus

18. _____ Palmaris longus

19. _____ Pronator quadratus

20. _____ Pronator teres

21. _____ Supinator

A. Base of first distal phalange, dorsal side

B. Base of first proximal phalange, dorsal side

C. Base of second and third metacarpals, palmar side

D. Base of third metacarpal, dorsal side

E. Base of fifth metacarpal, dorsal side

F. Base of fifth proximal phalange, dorsal side

G. Base of first distal phalange, palmar side

H. Bases of distal phalanges 2–5, palmar side

I. Distal one-fourth of medial side and anterior surface of ulna

J. Distal one-third of lateral supracondylar ridge

K. Flexor retinaculum and palmar aponeurosis

L. Lateral aspect of olecranon process and proximal posterior surface of ulna

M. Lateral side of radial styloid process

N. Middle one-third of lateral radius

O. Middle one-third of posterior surface of ulna, radius, and interosseous membrane

P. Middle and distal phalanges 2–5

Q. Pisiform, hook of hamate, and base of fifth metacarpal, palmar side

R. Posterior surface of body of ulna and interosseous membrane

S. Proximal one-third of posterior, lateral, and anterior surfaces of radius

T. Sides of middle phalanges 2–5

U. Tuberosity and coronoid process of ulna

LABEL JOINTS AND LIGAMENTS

This next activity will help you explore the joints of the elbow, forearm, wrist, and hand and the ligaments that hold them together.

INSTRUCTIONS. Label the bones and ligaments of the elbow, forearm, wrist, and hand.

List of Structures, Elbow and Forearm, Anterior View

Annular ligament	Medial epicondyle	Ulna
Humeroulnar joint capsule	Oblique cord	Ulnar collateral ligament
Humerus	Radial collateral ligament	
Interosseous membrane	Radius	

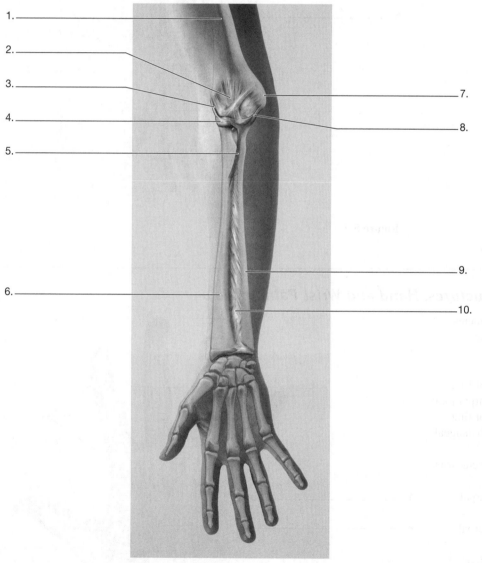

1.

2.

3.

4.

5.

6.

7.

8.

9.

10.

Figure 5.8

List of Structures, Elbow and Forearm, Posterior View

Annular ligament
Interosseous membrane
Lateral epicondyle
Medial epicondyle
Olecranon fossa
Olecranon process
Radial collateral
    ligament
Radial head
Radius
Ulna
Ulnar ridge

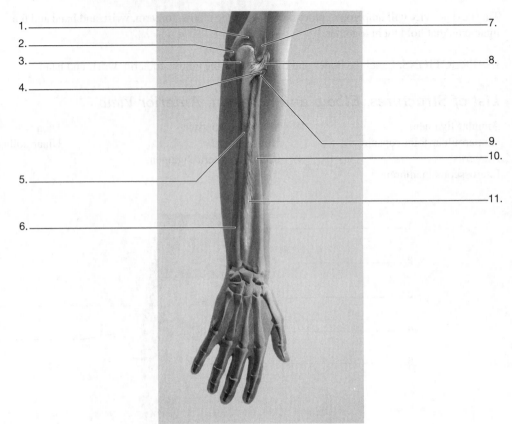

Figure 5.9

List of Structures, Hand and Wrist Palmar View

Collateral ligaments
Deep transverse
    metacarpal
    ligaments
Joint capsule of first
    carpometacarpal joint
Joint capsule of first
    metacarpophalangeal
    joint
Palmar carpometacarpal
    ligaments
Palmar metacarpal
    ligaments
Palmar radiocarpal
    ligament
Palmar radioulnar
    ligament
Palmar ulnocarpal
    ligament

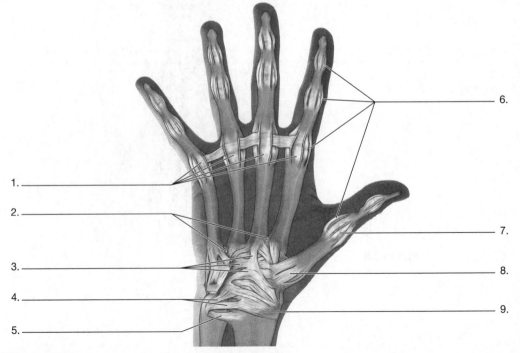

Figure 5.10

COMPLETE THE TABLE

This activity will help you study the function of ligaments of the elbow, forearm, wrist, and hand.

INSTRUCTIONS. Fill in the missing information. The first column indicates a ligament of this region, the second identifies which bony landmarks it joins, and the third indicates the function of the ligament or what movements are limited by this structure. The first one is completed for you as an example.

Ligament	Bony Landmarks Joined	Function
Annular	Radial head Proximal ulna	Stabilizes proximal radioulnar joint as forearm pronates and supinates
Collateral		
Deep transverse metacarpal		
Interosseous membrane		
Palmar carpometacarpal		
Palmar metacarpal		
Palmar radiocarpal		
Palmar radioulnar		
Palmar ulnocarpal		
Radial collateral		
Ulnar collateral		

LABEL MUSCLES OF THE ELBOW, FOREARM, WRIST, AND HAND

The following activities will help you learn to identify the muscles of the elbow, forearm, wrist, and hand.

INSTRUCTIONS. The following diagrams depict the superficial muscles and other important tissues of the elbow, forearm, wrist, and hand. Label each of the following structures.

List of Structures, Anterior View

Biceps brachii
Bicipital aponeurosis
Brachialis (use twice)
Brachioradialis
Extensor carpi radialis brevis
Extensor carpi radialis longus

Flexor carpi radialis
Flexor carpi ulnaris
Flexor digitorum profundus
Flexor digitorum superficialis
Flexor pollicis longus
Flexor retinaculum

Palmar aponeurosis
Palmaris longus
Pronator quadratus
Pronator teres

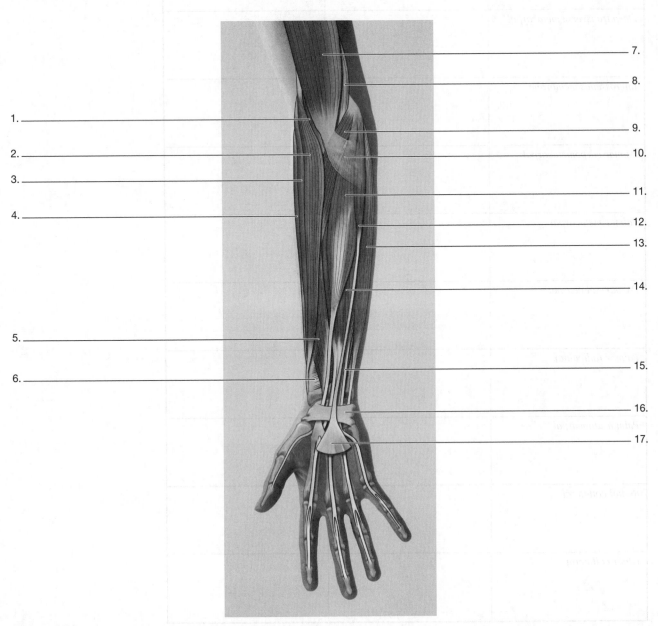

Figure 5.11

List of Structures, Posterior View

Abductor pollicis longus
Anconeus
Brachioradialis
Extensor carpi radialis brevis
Extensor carpi radialis longus

Extensor carpi ulnaris
Extensor digiti minimi
Extensor digitorum
Extensor indices
Extensor pollicis brevis

Extensor pollicis longus
Flexor carpi ulnaris
Triceps brachii (lateral head)
Triceps brachii (medial head)

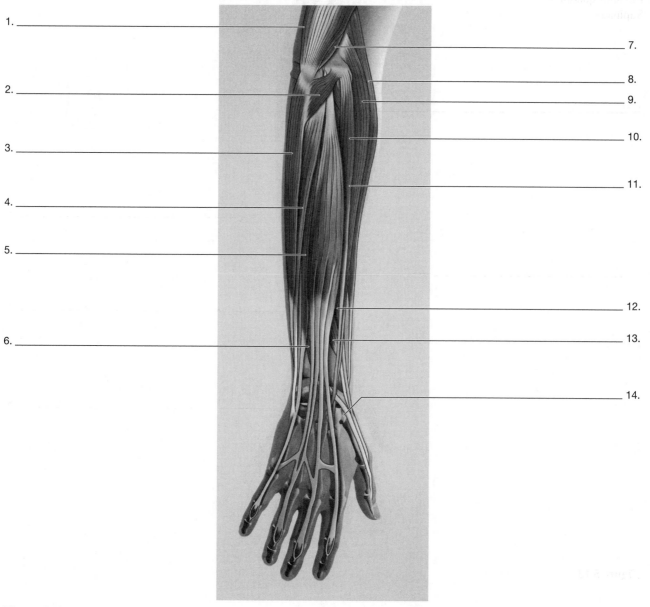

1. _____

2. _____

3. _____

4. _____

5. _____

6. _____

7. _____

8. _____

9. _____

10. _____

11. _____

12. _____

13. _____

14. _____

Figure 5.12

INSTRUCTIONS. The following diagrams depict the deep muscles of the elbow, forearm, wrist, and hand. Color and label each of the following structures.

List of Structures, Anterior View

Flexor digitorum profundus
Flexor pollicis longus
Lumbricals
Pronator quadratus
Supinator

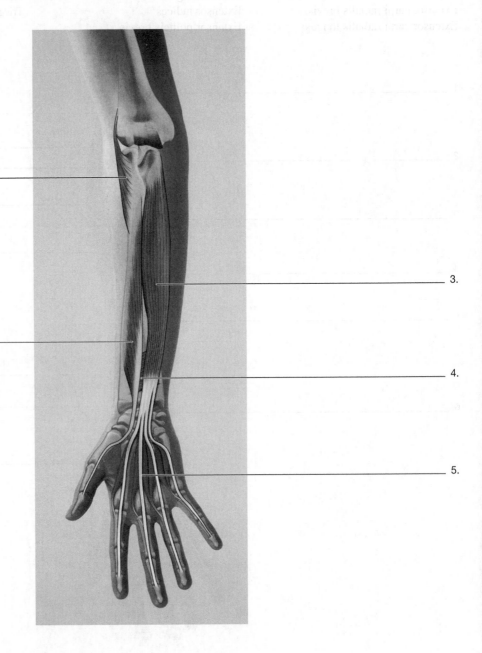

1. _____

2. _____

3. _____

4. _____

5. _____

Figure 5.13

List of Structures, Posterior View

Abductor pollicis longus
Anconeus
Extensor indicis
Extensor pollicis brevis
Extensor pollicis longus
Supinator

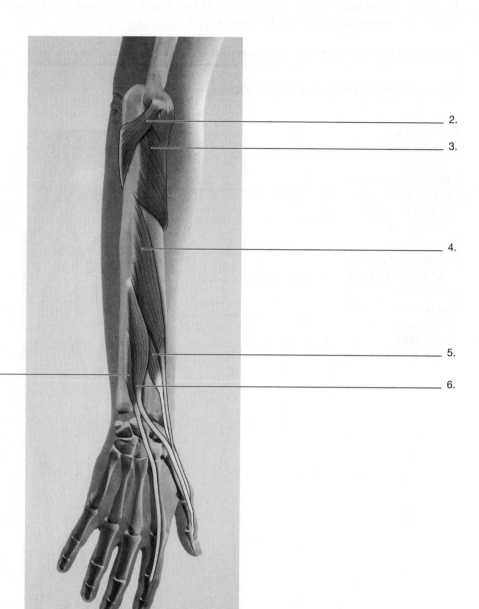

Figure 5.14

LABEL SPECIAL STRUCTURES

This exercise will help you become aware of blood vessels, lymph nodes and vessels, and nerves when palpating and working in this area.

INSTRUCTIONS. Label the following special structures of the elbow, forearm, wrist, and hand.

List of Structures, Anterior View

Basilic vein
Brachial artery
Cephalic vein
    (use twice)
Cubital lymph nodes
Medial cubital vein
Medial epicondyle
    of humerus
Median nerve
Palmar and digital
    arteries and nerves
Radial artery
Radial nerve
Ulnar artery
Ulnar nerve
    (use twice)

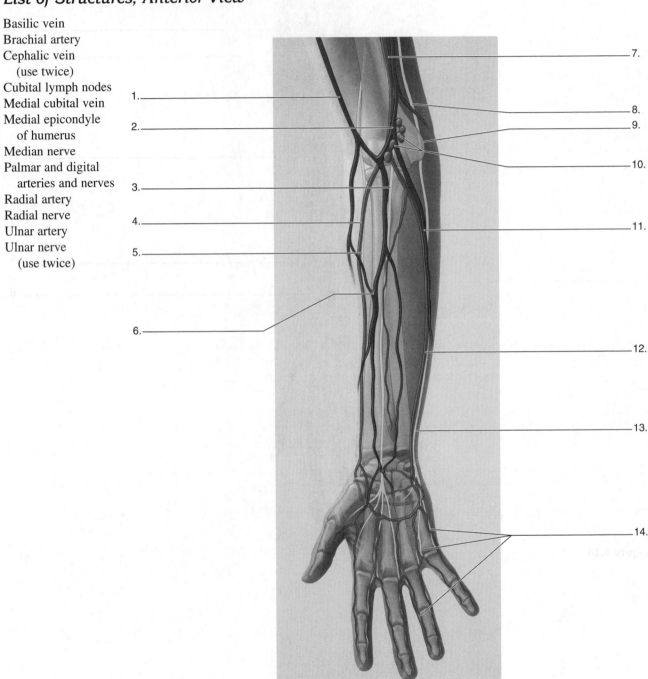

Figure 5.15

List of Structures, Posterior View

Anconeus

Cubital notch

Extensor carpi ulnaris

Flexor carpi ulnaris

Humerus

Radial nerve

Olecranon process

Posterior ulnar recurrent artery

Recurrent interosseous artery

Ulnar nerve

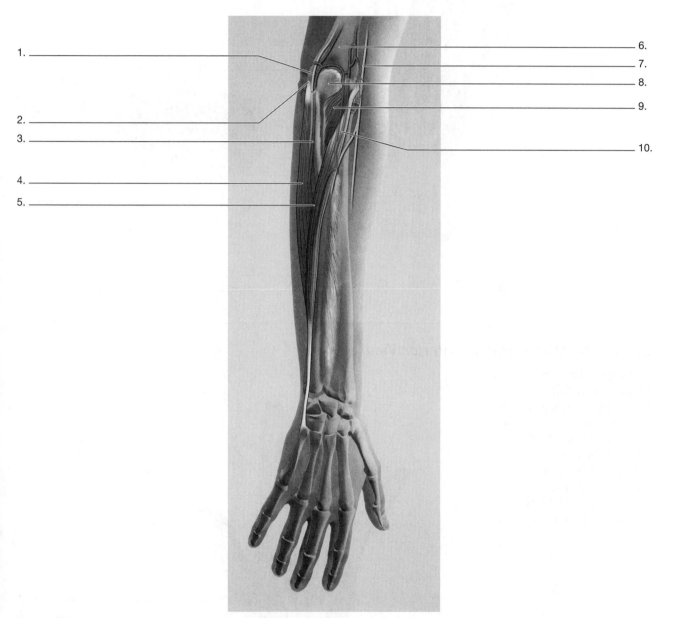

1.

2.

3.

4.

5.

6.

7.

8.

9.

10.

Figure 5.16

List of Structures, Carpal Tunnel

Carpal bones
Finger flexor
    tendons (use twice)
Flexor retinaculum
    (use twice)
Median nerve
    (use twice)

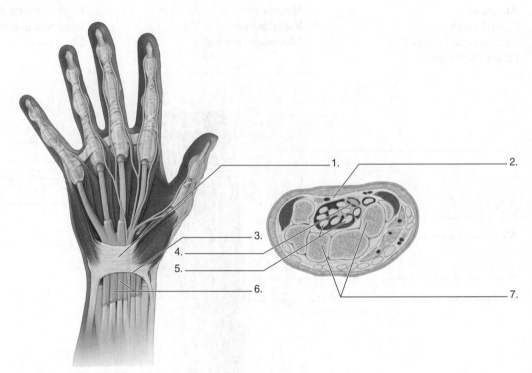

Figure 5.17

List of Structures, Hand, Anterior View

Abductor pollicis brevis
Flexor carpi radialis
Flexor digitorum superficialis
    and profundus in common
    flexor synovial sheath
Flexor pollicis brevis
Flexor pollicis longus
Flexor retinaculum
Flexor tendons of the fingers
    and hand in synovial sheaths

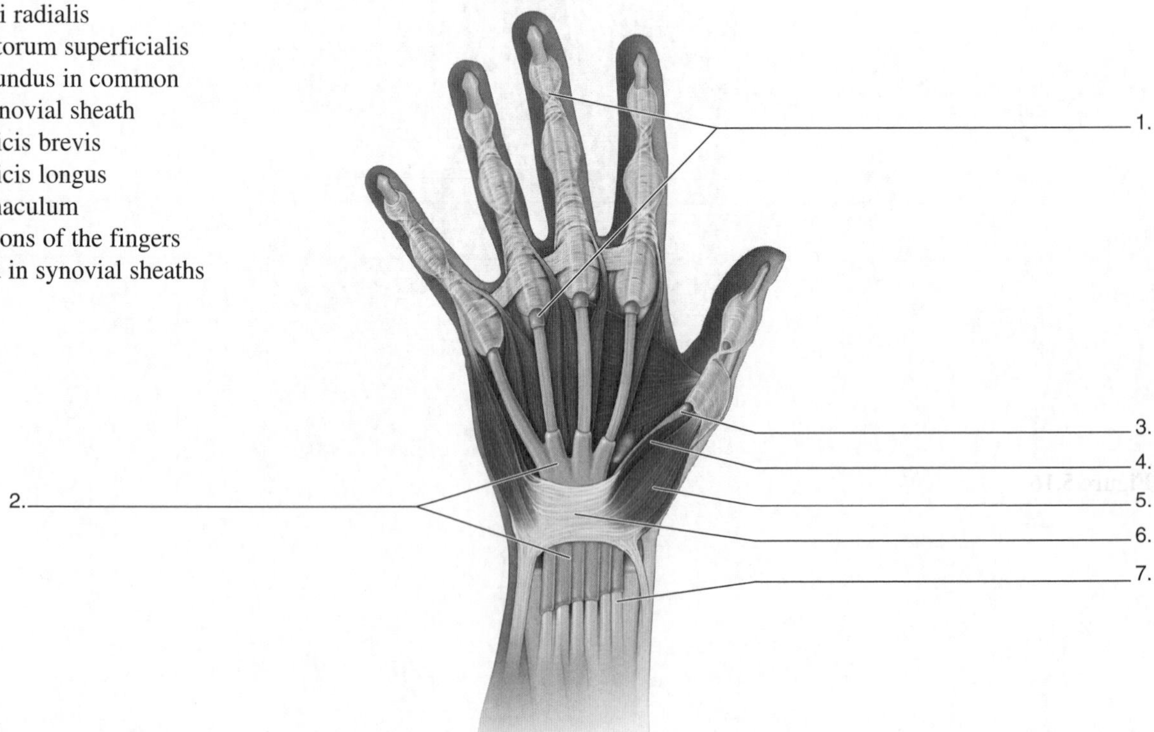

Figure 5.18

IDENTIFY MOVEMENTS OF THE ELBOW, FOREARM, WRIST, AND HAND

In this activity, you will identify the individual motions of the elbow, forearm, wrist, and hand. This will help you appreciate how these movements are created.

INSTRUCTIONS. Beneath each of the following figures, write the name of each motion.

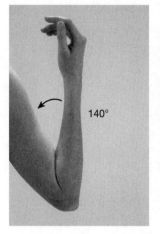 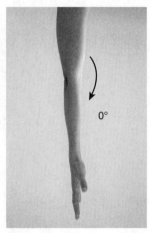 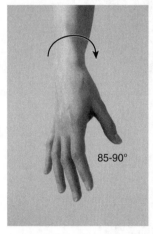 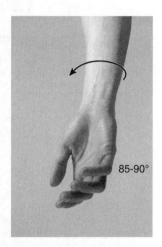

1._____ 2._____ 3._____ 4._____

Figure 5.19

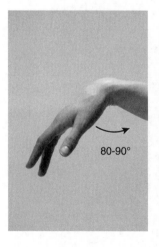 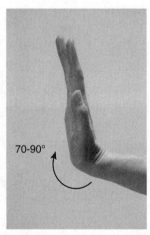 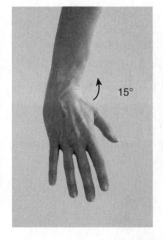 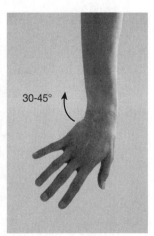

1._____ 2._____ 3._____ 4._____

Figure 5.20

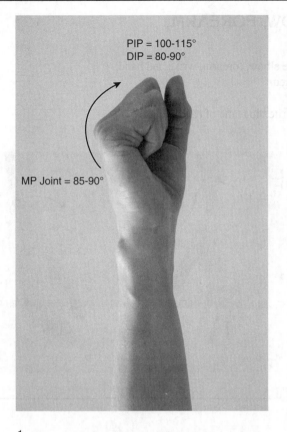

PIP = 100-115°
DIP = 80-90°

MP Joint = 85-90°

1. _____

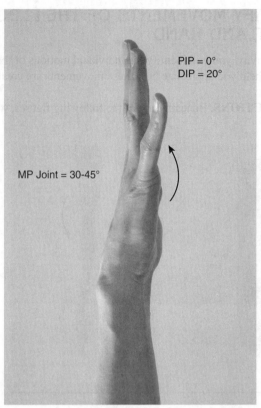

PIP = 0°
DIP = 20°

MP Joint = 30-45°

2. _____

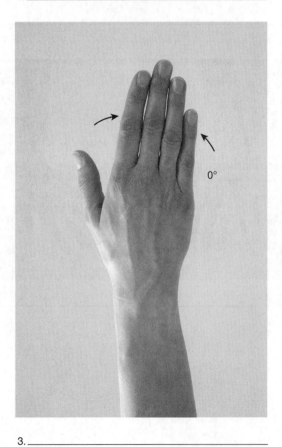

0°

3. _____

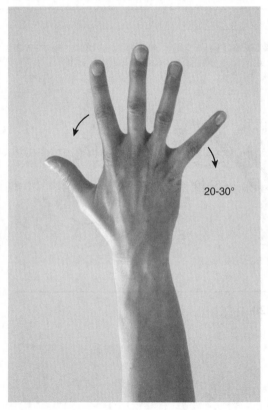

20-30°

4. _____

Figure 5.21

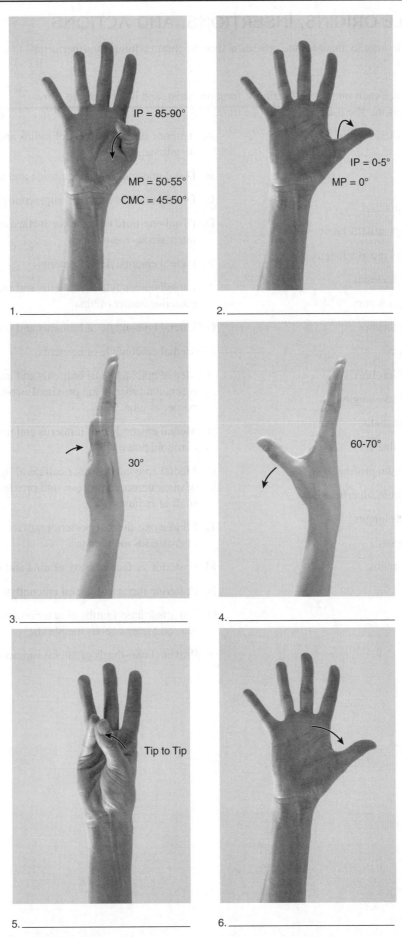

1. _____

IP = 85-90°

MP = 50-55°
CMC = 45-50°

2. _____

IP = 0-5°
MP = 0°

3. _____

30°

4. _____

60-70°

5. _____

Tip to Tip

6. _____

Figure 5.22

MATCH MUSCLE ORIGINS, INSERTIONS, AND ACTIONS

Each muscle has unique muscle attachments, crosses a specific joint or joints, and performs specific movements.

INSTRUCTIONS. Match each muscle of the elbow, forearm, wrist, and hand with the corresponding origin. Answers may be used more than one time.

1. _____ Abductor pollicis longus

2. _____ Anconeus

3. _____ Brachialis

4. _____ Brachioradialis

5. _____ Extensor carpi radialis brevis

6. _____ Extensor carpi radialis longus

7. _____ Extensor carpi ulnaris

8. _____ Extensor digiti minimi

9. _____ Extensor digitorum

10. _____ Extensor indicis

11. _____ Extensor pollicis brevis

12. _____ Extensor pollicis longus

13. _____ Flexor carpi radialis

14. _____ Flexor carpi ulnaris

15. _____ Flexor digitorum profundus

16. _____ Flexor digitorum superficialis

17. _____ Flexor pollicis longus

18. _____ Palmaris longus

19. _____ Pronator quadratus

20. _____ Pronator teres

21. _____ Supinator

A. Anterior surface of body of radius and interosseous membrane

B. Distal one-fourth of medial side and anterior surface of ulna

C. Distal one-third of lateral supracondylar ridge

D. Distal one-third of posterior surface of radius and interosseous membrane

E. Lateral epicondyle of humerus

F. Lateral epicondyle of humerus and middle one-third of posterior border of ulna

G. Lateral epicondyle of humerus and supinator crest of ulna

H. Medial epicondyle of humerus

I. Medial epicondyle of humerus and medial aspect of olecranon process and proximal two-thirds of the lateral border of ulna

J. Medial epicondyle of humerus and medial aspect of ulnar coronoid process

K. Medial epicondyle, ulnar collateral ligament, medial aspect of ulnar coronoid process, and proximal one-half of anterior shaft of radius

L. Middle one-third of posterior surface of ulna, radius, and interosseous membrane

M. Posterior surface of body of ulna and interosseous membrane

N. Posterior surface of lateral epicondyle

O. Proximal three-fourths of anterior and medial surfaces of ulna and interosseous membrane

P. Proximal two-thirds of lateral supracondylar ridge

INSTRUCTIONS. Match each muscle of elbow, forearm, wrist, and hand with the corresponding insertion. Use each answer one time.

1. _____ Abductor pollicis longus

2. _____ Anconeus

3. _____ Brachialis

4. _____ Brachioradialis

5. _____ Extensor carpi radialis brevis

6. _____ Extensor carpi radialis longus

7. _____ Extensor carpi ulnaris

8. _____ Extensor digiti minimi

9. _____ Extensor digitorum

10. _____ Extensor indicis

11. _____ Extensor pollicis brevis

12. _____ Extensor pollicis longus

13. _____ Flexor carpi radialis

14. _____ Flexor carpi ulnaris

15. _____ Flexor digitorum profundus

16. _____ Flexor digitorum superficialis

17. _____ Flexor pollicis longus

18. _____ Palmaris longus

19. _____ Pronator quadratus

20. _____ Pronator teres

21. _____ Supinator

A. Base of first distal phalange, dorsal side

B. Base of first distal phalange, palmar side

C. Base of first metacarpal, dorsal side

D. Base of first proximal phalange, dorsal side

E. Base of second and third metacarpals, palmar side

F. Base of second metacarpal, dorsal side

G. Base of second proximal phalange and into tendon of extensor digitorum

H. Base of third metacarpal, dorsal side

I. Base of fifth metacarpal, dorsal side

J. Base of fifth proximal phalange, dorsal side

K. Base of distal phalanges 2–5, palmar side by four separate tendons

L. Distal one-fourth of radius on lateral side and anterior surface

M. Flexor retinaculum and palmar aponeurosis

N. Lateral aspect of olecranon process and proximal posterior surface of body of ulna

O. Lateral side of radial styloid process

P. Middle one-third of lateral radius

Q. Middle and distal phalanges 2–5, dorsal side

R. Pisiform, hook of hamate, and base of fifth metacarpal on palmar side

S. Proximal one-third of posterior, lateral, and anterior surfaces of radius

T. Sides of middle phalanges 2–5 by four separate tendons

U. Tuberosity and coronoid process of ulna

INSTRUCTIONS. Match each muscle of the elbow, forearm, wrist, and hand with the corresponding actions. Choose all that apply. Some answers will be used more than once.

1. _____ Abductor pollicis longus

2. _____ Anconeus

3. _____ Brachialis

4. _____ Brachioradialis

5. _____ Extensor carpi radialis brevis

6. _____ Extensor carpi radialis longus

7. _____ Extensor carpi ulnaris

8. _____ Extensor digiti minimi

9. _____ Extensor digitorum

10. _____ Extensor indicis

11. _____ Extensor pollicis brevis

12. _____ Extensor pollicis longus

13. _____ Flexor carpi radialis

14. _____ Flexor carpi ulnaris

15. _____ Flexor digitorum profundus

16. _____ Flexor digitorum superficialis

17. _____ Flexor pollicis longus

18. _____ Palmaris longus

19. _____ Pronator quadratus

20. _____ Pronator teres

21. _____ Supinator

A. Elbow extension

B. Elbow flexion

C. Finger abduction

D. Finger adduction

E. Finger extension

F. Finger flexion

G. Pronation

H. Radial deviation

I. Supination

J. Thumb abduction

K. Thumb adduction

L. Thumb extension

M. Thumb flexion

N. Thumb opposition

O. Ulnar deviation

P. Wrist extension

Q. Wrist flexion

IDENTIFY SHORTENING AND LENGTHENING MUSCLES

For each of the following muscles, identify the position where the muscle is most shortened and the position that lengthens or stretches the muscle. (Hint: Moving into the muscle actions will shorten and reversing them will lengthen or stretch.) The first one is completed as an example.

Abductor Pollicis Longus

Shortened position: Extend and abduct the first carpometacarpal joint, and flex and radially deviate the wrist.

Lengthened position: Flex and adduct the first carpometacarpal joint, and extend and ulnar deviate the wrist.

Brachioradialis

Shortened position: _____

_____

_____

Lengthened position: _____

_____

_____

Extensor Carpi Radialis Longus

Shortened position: _____

_____

_____

Lengthened position: _____

_____

_____

Extensor Carpi Ulnaris

Shortened position: _____

_____

_____

Lengthened position: _____

_____

_____

Extensor Digitorum

Shortened position: _____

_____

_____

Lengthened position: _____

_____

_____

Flexor Carpi Radialis

Shortened position: _____

_____

_____

Lengthened position: _____

_____

_____

Flexor Carpi Ulnaris

Shortened position: _____

_____

_____

Lengthened position: _____

_____

_____

Flexor Digitorum Profundus

Shortened position: _____

_____

_____

Lengthened position: _____

_____

_____

Palmaris Longus

Shortened position: _____

_____

_____

Lengthened position: _____

_____

_____

Pronator Teres

Shortened position: _____

_____

_____

Lengthened position: _____

_____

_____

COMPLETE THE TABLE: SYNERGISTS/ANTAGONISTS

This activity will help you gain a better sense of how the muscles of the elbow, forearm, wrist, and hand work together or in opposition.

INSTRUCTIONS. Fill in the missing information about muscles of the elbow, forearm, wrist, and hand. The first column indicates a movement of the shoulder, the second identifies which muscles perform this action, and the third indicates the opposite action. The first one is completed for you as an example.

Movement	Muscles	Opposite Action
Elbow extension	Anconeus Extensor carpi ulnaris Extensor digiti minimi Extensor digitorum Supinator Triceps brachii	Elbow flexion
Elbow flexion		
Finger abduction		
Finger adduction		
Finger extension		
Finger flexion		
Pronation		
Radial deviation		

(*Continued on next page*)

Movement	Muscles	Opposite Action
Supination		
Thumb abduction		
Thumb adduction		
Thumb extension		
Thumb flexion		
Thumb opposition		
Ulnar deviation		
Wrist extension		
Wrist flexion		

PUTTING THE ELBOW, FOREARM, WRIST, AND HAND IN MOTION

The following activity brings together all that you have learned about the elbow, forearm, wrist, and hand. As you did in the previous chapter on the shoulder, you will examine several specific movements. For each movement, you will describe: (1) which joints are involved, (2) which joint motions occur, and (3) in what sequence these occur. It is often helpful to perform the movement yourself, observe someone else performing the movement, or watch an animation or video of the movement to better understand what is happening and when.

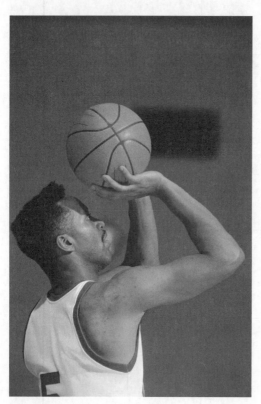

Figure 5.23 Basketball free throw

INSTRUCTIONS. List the joints involved in the movement shown.

_____

_____

_____

INSTRUCTIONS. List the motions that occur at each joint.

_____

_____

_____

INSTRUCTIONS. List the sequence of events involved in the movement shown.

_____

_____

_____

_____

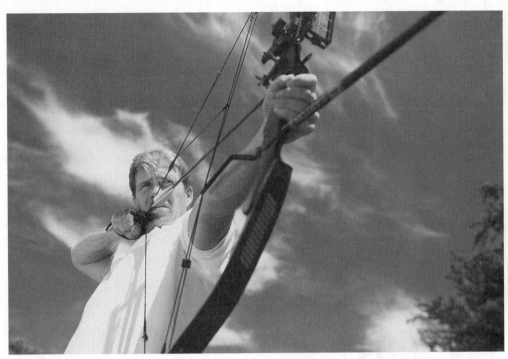

Figure 5.24 Drawing a bow

INSTRUCTIONS. List the joints involved in the movement shown.

_____

_____

_____

INSTRUCTIONS. List the motions that occur at each joint.

_____

_____

_____

INSTRUCTIONS. List the sequence of events involved in the movement shown.

_____

_____

_____

_____

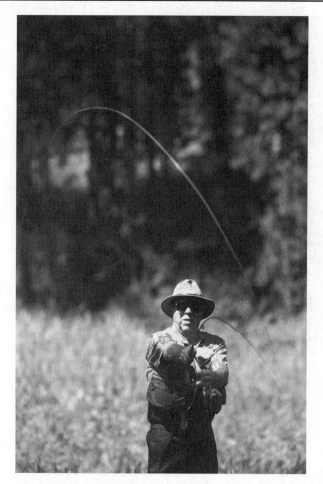

Figure 5.25 Casting a line.

INSTRUCTIONS. List the joints involved in the movement shown.

_____

_____

_____

INSTRUCTIONS. List the motions that occur at each joint.

_____

_____

_____

INSTRUCTIONS. List the sequence of events involved in the movement shown.

_____

_____

_____

_____

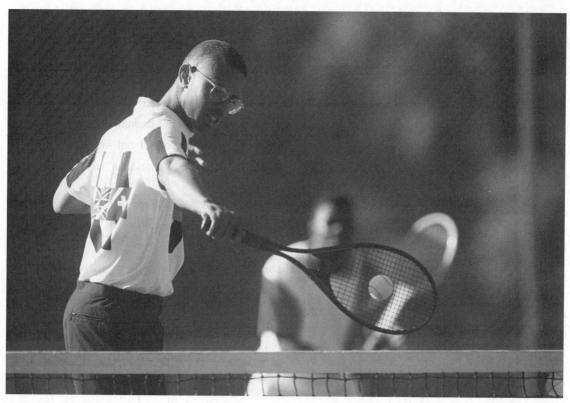

Figure 5.26 Tennis forehand

INSTRUCTIONS. List the joints involved in the movement shown.

_____

_____

_____

INSTRUCTIONS. List the motions that occur at each joint.

_____

_____

_____

INSTRUCTIONS. List the sequence of events involved in the movement shown.

_____

_____

_____

_____

WORD CHALLENGE

This final exercise checks your recall of terms and concepts introduced throughout the chapter.

INSTRUCTIONS. Complete the crossword using the following clues.

ACROSS:

4. Number of interphalangeal joints in the thumb.
5. Lateral long bone of the forearm in anatomical position.
7. Medial long bone of the forearm in anatomical position.
10. Elbow flexor.
12. Number of carpal bones.
14. Connects the medial radius to the tuberosity of the ulna.

DOWN:

1. Assists triceps brachii in extending the elbow.
2. The most lateral of the superficial wrist flexors.
3. Passageway containing the median nerve and flexor tendons of the fingers and thumb.
6. Anatomical depression formed by tendons in the hand.
8. Carpal bone distal to the scaphoid.
9. Each finger has three.
11. To rotate the forearm to cause the palm to face anteriorly.
13. Its hook can be palpated distally to the pisiform.

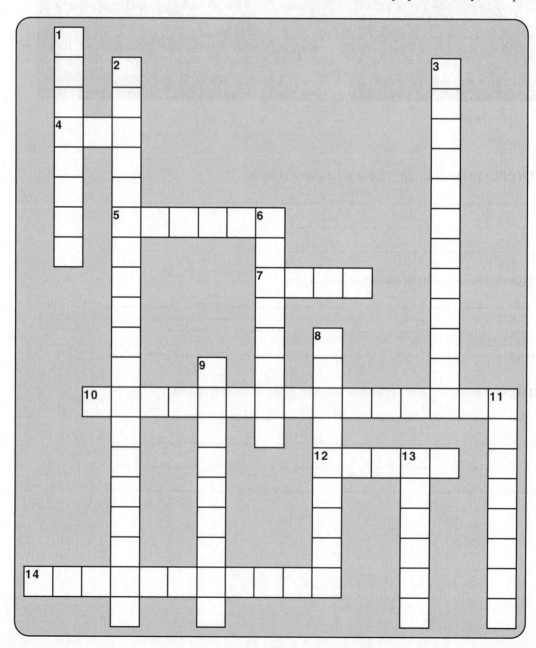

Head, Neck, and Face

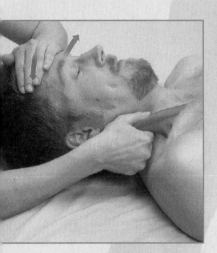

We begin our exploration of the axial skeleton with the head, neck, and face. Seven delicate cervical vertebrae are stacked on top of the stable rib cage. The skull rests on the atlas (C1) and contains the brain and several sensory organs. Twenty-six individual bones form the skull. The mandible connects with the skull to form the jaw, a complex structure capable of movement in multiple directions. The activities in this chapter will help increase your understanding of the structure and function of the head, neck, and face.

LABEL SURFACE LANDMARKS

Because so many delicate structures are located in the head, neck, and face, it is especially important to orient yourself during palpation. Several significant surface landmarks are helpful with this process. The following activities will help to familiarize you with them.

INSTRUCTIONS. The following images depict the major surface landmarks of the head, neck, and face. Label and color each of the following in the spaces provided.

List of Structures, Anterior View

Clavicle	Mental protuberance	Trapezius
Frontal eminence	Supraorbital margin	Zygomatic bone
Mandible	Thyroid cartilage	

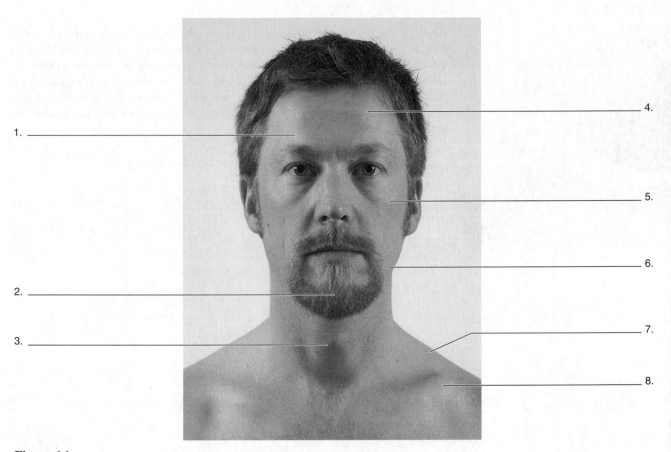

Figure 6.1

List of Structures, Posterior View

External occipital
   protuberance
Mastoid process
Nuchal ligament

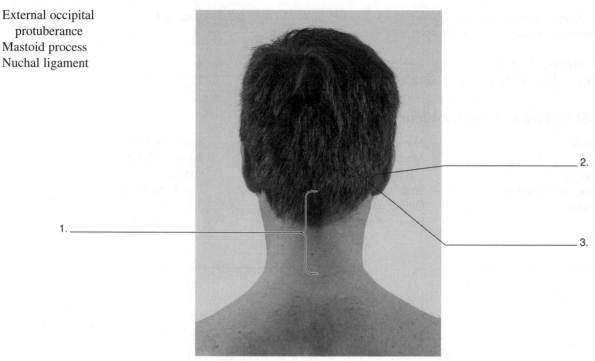

Figure 6.2

List of Structures, Anterolateral View

Angle of mandible
Anterior triangle
Clavicle
External occipital protuberance

Mastoid process
Mental protuberance
Posterior triangle
Sternocleidomastoid muscle

Temporal fossa
Thyroid cartilage
Trapezius

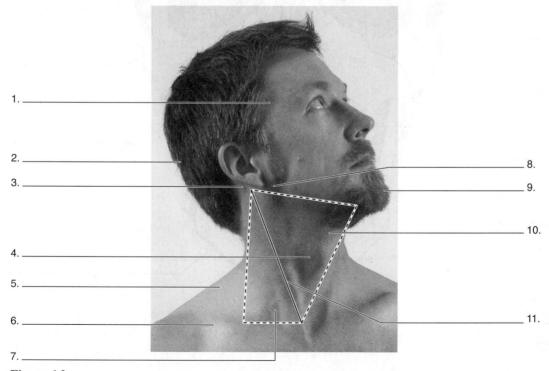

Figure 6.3

COLOR AND LABEL SKELETAL STRUCTURES

Bones and bony landmarks provide consistent touchstones as we locate, differentiate, and explore soft-tissue structures such as muscles, tendons, and ligaments.

INSTRUCTIONS. The following images depict the bones and bony landmarks for the head, neck, and face. Color and label each of the following structures.

List of Structures, Anterior View

Cranial sutures	Maxilla	Sphenoid bone
Ethmoid bone	Mental protuberance	Temporal bone
Frontal bone	Nasal bones	Vomer
Greater wing of sphenoid bone	Nasal cavity	Zygomatic bone
Lacrimal bone	Orbital cavity	
Mandible	Parietal bone	

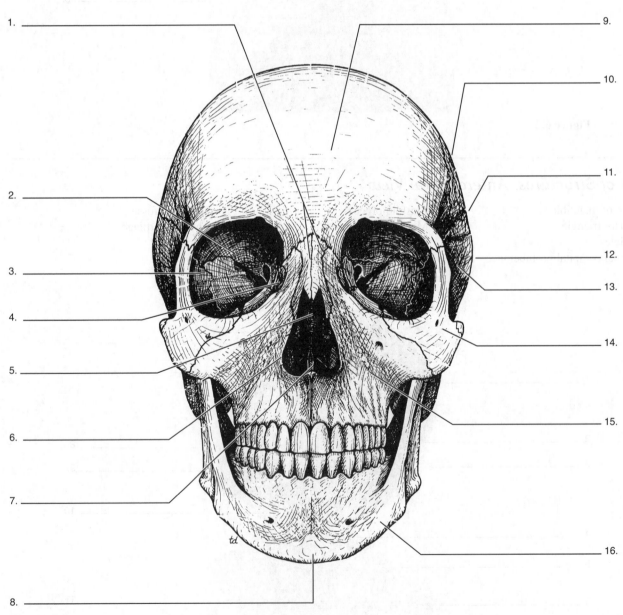

Figure 6.4

List of Structures, Inferior View

Basilar part of occipital bone
External occipital
  protuberance
Foramen magnum
Inferior nuchal line
Mandibular fossa
Maxilla

Occipital bone
Occipital condyles
Palatine bone
Palatine process of maxilla
Parietal bone
Pterygoid plates
Sphenoid bone

Styloid process
Superior nuchal line
Temporal bone
Vomer
Zygomatic bone
Zygomatic process of the
  temporal bone

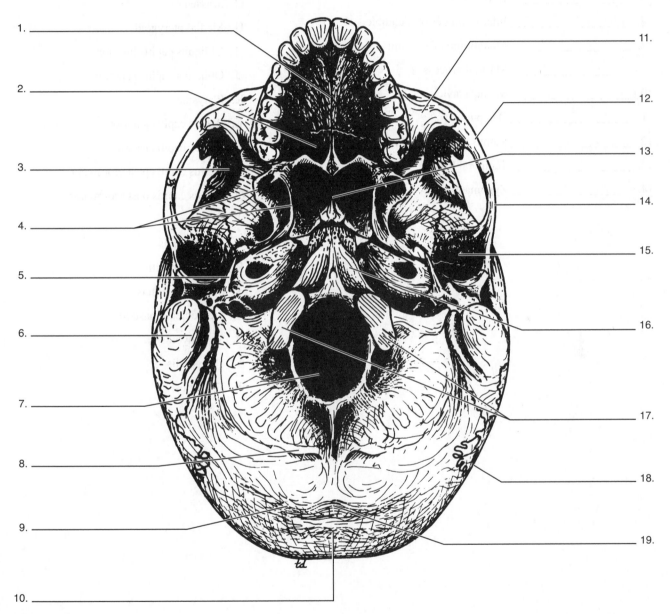

1.
2.
3.
4.
5.
6.
7.
8.
9.
10.

11.
12.
13.
14.
15.
16.
17.
18.
19.

Figure 6.5

INSTRUCTIONS. Match each of the following bony landmarks with the corresponding muscle of the head, neck, and face. Choose all that apply. Some answers will be used more than once.

1. _____ Anterior bodies of cervical vertebra

2. _____ Cervical spinous processes

3. _____ Cervical transverse processes

4. _____ Coronoid process of mandible

5. _____ First and second rib

6. _____ Hyoid bone

7. _____ Inferior border of mandible

8. _____ Manubrium of sternum

9. _____ Mastoid process

10. _____ Medial clavicle

11. _____ Occiput

12. _____ Ramus and angle of mandible

13. _____ Temporal fossa

14. _____ Zygomatic arch

A. Digastric

B. Infrahyoids

C. Lateral pterygoid

D. Levator scapulae

E. Longus capitis

F. Longus colli

G. Masseter

H. Medial pterygoid

I. Obliquus capitis inferior

J. Obliquus capitis superior

K. Platysma

L. Rectus capitis anterior

M. Rectus capitis lateralis

N. Rectus capitis posterior major

O. Rectus capitis posterior minor

P. Scalenes

Q. Semispinalis

R. Splenius capitis

S. Splenius cervicis

T. Sternocleidomastoid

U. Suprahyoids

V. Temporalis

W. Trapezius

LABEL JOINTS AND LIGAMENTS

The next activities explore the joints of the head, neck, and face and the ligaments that hold them together.

INSTRUCTIONS. The following images depict the bones and ligaments of the head, neck, and face. Color and label the following structures.

List of Structures, Deep Posterior View

Alar ligaments   Axis   Ligamenta flava
Atlas   Cruciate ligament   Transverse ligament

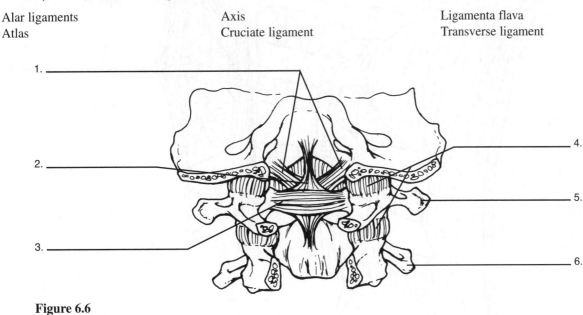

Figure 6.6

List of Structures, Intermediate Posterior View

Atlas   Occiput   Tectorial membrane (deep portions)
Axis   Posterior longitudinal ligament Tectorial membrane

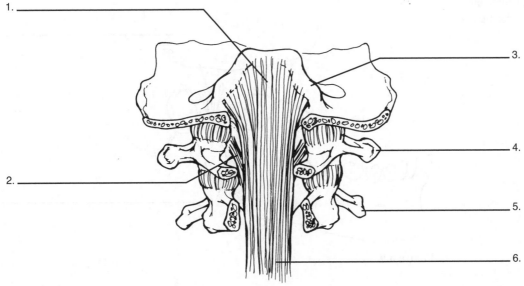

Figure 6.7

List of Structures, Lateral View

Interspinal ligaments
Ligamenta flava
Ligamentum nuchae

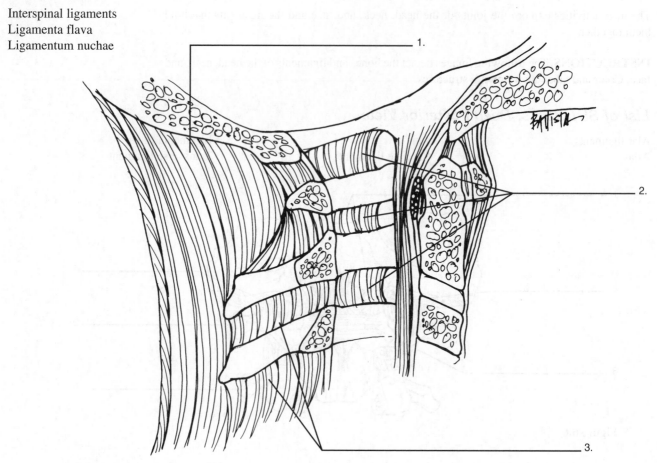

1.

2.

3.

Figure 6.8

List of Structures, Jaw Lateral View

Stylomandibular ligament
Temporomandibular ligament

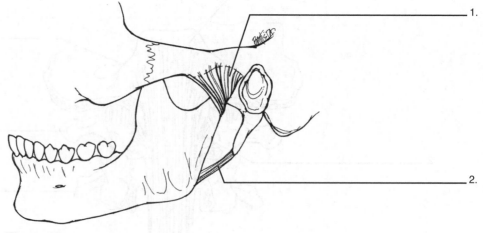

1.

2.

Figure 6.9

COMPLETE THE TABLE: LIGAMENTS

This activity will help you review the functions of the various ligaments.

INSTRUCTIONS. Fill in the missing information regarding ligaments of the head, neck, and face. The first column indicates a ligament of this region, the second identifies which bony landmarks it joins, and the third indicates the function of the ligament or which movements are limited by this structure. The first one is completed for you as an example.

Ligament	Bony Landmarks Joined	Function
Alar	Occiput Atlas	Limit rotation of atlanto-occipital joint
Anterior atlantoaxial		
Anterior atlanto-occipital		
Anterior longitudinal		
Cruciate		
Interspinal		
Ligamentum flavum		
Ligamentum nuchae		
Posterior atlantoaxial		
Posterior atlanto-occipital		

(Continued on next page)

Ligament	Bony Landmarks Joined	Function
Posterior longitudinal		
Sphenomandibular		
Stylomandibular		
Tectorial		
Temporomandibular		
Transverse ligament of axis		

LABEL MUSCLES OF THE HEAD, NECK, AND FACE

In the following exercises, you'll label the muscles of the head, neck, and face in layers. Superficial muscles protect underlying structures; position the head, neck, and shoulder; and affect the entire upper body. Intermediate muscles produce movements and anchor head position. Deep muscles fix one vertebra to another, stabilize the skull on the atlas, fine-tune head position, and maintain balanced posture of the head and neck. Specialized muscles facilitate chewing, speech, and facial expressions.

INSTRUCTIONS. The following diagrams depict the superficial muscles of the head, neck, and face. Label each of the following structures.

List of Structures, Anterolateral View

Anterior scalene
Levator scapula
Middle scalene

Omohyoid
Posterior scalene
Splenius capitis

Sternocleidomastoid
Trapezius

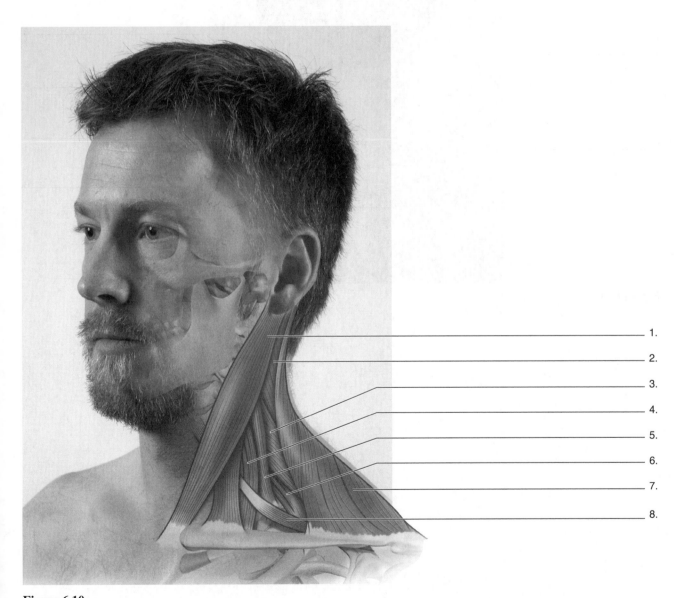

1. _____

2. _____

3. _____

4. _____

5. _____

6. _____

7. _____

8. _____

Figure 6.10

List of Structures, Posterior View

Levator scapula   Splenius capitis   Sternocleidomastoid
Semispinalis capitis   Splenius cervicis   Trapezius

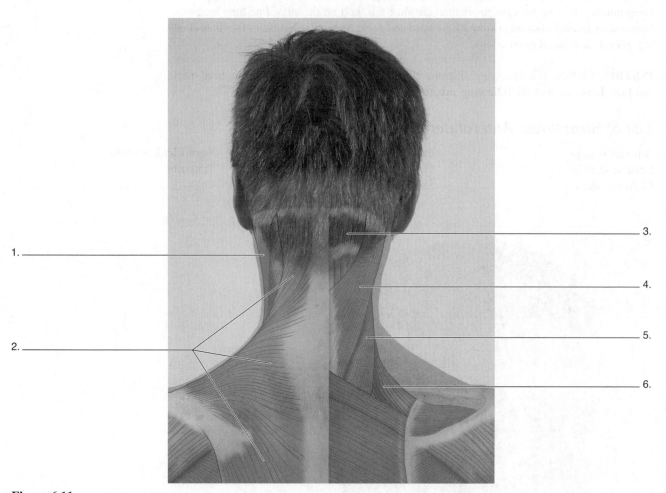

Figure 6.11

INSTRUCTIONS. The following diagrams depict the intermediate muscles of the head and neck. Label each of the following structures.

List of Structures, Anterior View

Digastric (use twice)
Geniohyoid
Mylohyoid
Omohyoid (use three times)
Sternocleidomastoid
Sternohyoid
Sternothyroid
Stylohyoid
Thyrohyoid
Trapezius

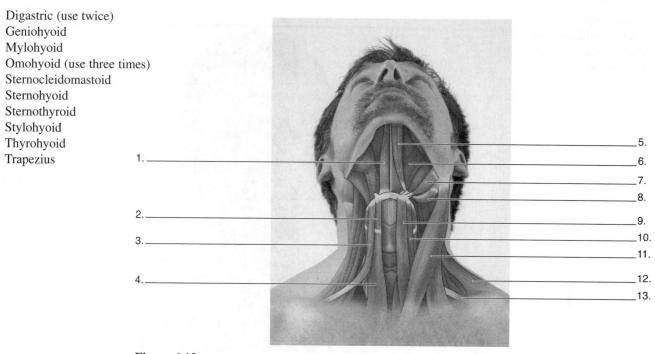

1. _____
2. _____
3. _____
4. _____

5. _____
6. _____
7. _____
8. _____
9. _____
10. _____
11. _____
12. _____
13. _____

Figure 6.12

List of Structures, Posterior View

Ligamentum nuchae
Splenius capitis
Splenius cervicis
Occiput
Semispinalis capitis
Middle scalene
Posterior scalene

1. _____
2. _____
3. _____

4. _____
5. _____
6. _____
7. _____

Figure 6.13

INSTRUCTIONS. The following diagrams depict the deep muscles of the head and neck. Label each of the following structures.

List of Structures, Anterior View

Longus capitis
Rectus capitis anterior
Rectus capitis lateralis
Longus colli

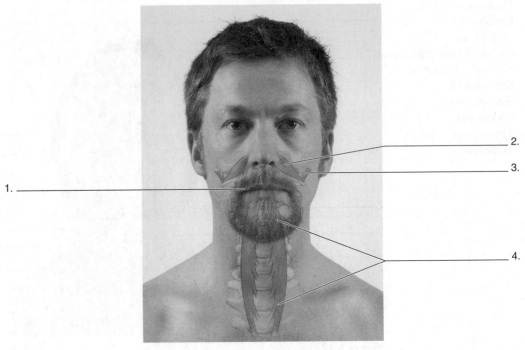

Figure 6.14

List of Structures, Posterior View

Longissimus capitis
Middle scalene
Multifidi
Obliquus capitis
    inferior
Obliquus capitis
    superior
Posterior scalene
Rectus capitis
    posterior minor
Rectus capitis
    posterior major
Rotatores (cervical)
Rotatores (thoracic)
Semispinalis
    cervicis

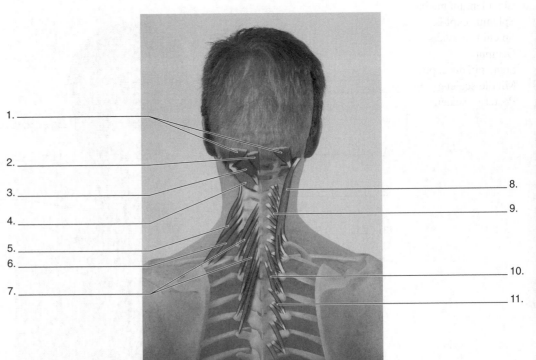

Figure 6.15

INSTRUCTIONS. The following diagram depicts the deep muscles of the face. Label each of the following structures:

List of Structures, Anterior View

Buccinator
Corrugator supercilii
Depressor anguli oris
Depressor labii inferioris
Frontalis
Galea aponeurotica

Levator labii superioris
Masseter
Mentalis
Nasalis
Orbicularis oculi (orbital)
Orbicularis oculi (palpebral)

Orbicularis oris
Platysma
Procerus
Risorius
Temporalis
Zygomaticus major and minor

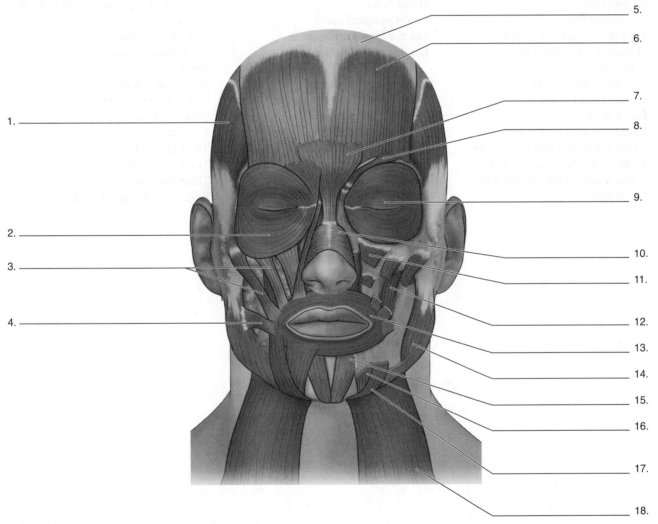

Figure 6.16

LABEL SPECIAL STRUCTURES

Several important structures are located in the head, neck, and face besides those directly responsible for movement. It is especially important that we are aware of blood vessels, lymph nodes and vessels, and nerves when palpating and working in this area.

INSTRUCTIONS. The following image depicts the special structures of the head, neck, and face. Use the following list to label each structure.

List of Structures, Superficial Anterolateral View

Accessory nerve
Anterior scalene muscle
Brachial plexus
Cervical plexus
Depressor anguli oris muscle
Depressor labii inferioris
    muscle
External carotid artery
External jugular vein
Facial artery
Facial nerve (buccal branch)
Facial nerve (mandibular branch)
Facial nerve (temporal branches)
Facial nerve (zygomatic branch)
Facial vein

Frontalis muscle
Great auricular nerve
Hyoid bone
Lesser occipital nerve
Levator anguli oris muscle
Levator labii superioris
    muscle
Levator scapula muscle
Mentalis muscle
Middle scalene muscle
Omohyoid muscle
Orbicularis oculi muscle
Orbicularis oris muscle
Parotid salivary gland
Procerus muscle

Sternocleidomastoid muscle
    (clavicular head)
Sternocleidomastoid muscle (sternal
    head)
Sternohyoid muscle
Sternothyroid muscle
Supraclavicular nerve
Supraorbital nerve
Supratrochlear nerve
Thyrohyoid muscle
Thyroid cartilage
Thyroid gland
Transverse colli nerve
Trapezius muscle
Zygomaticus major muscle

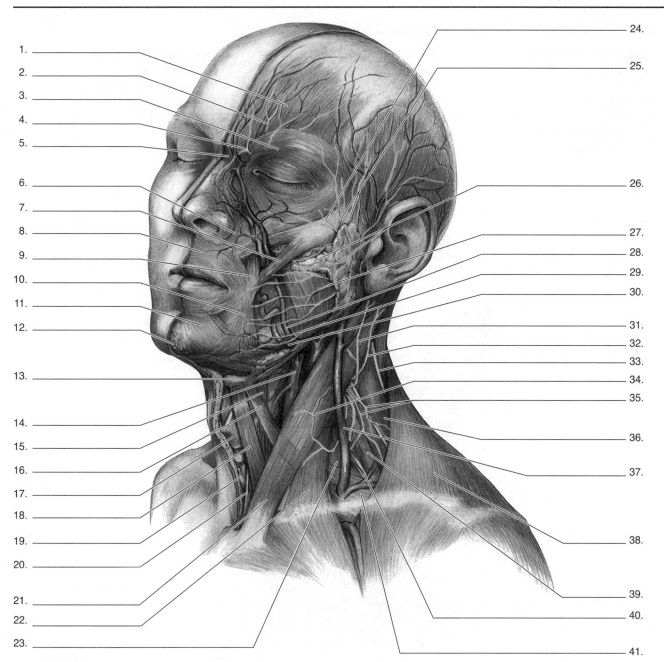

1. _____
2. _____
3. _____
4. _____
5. _____

6. _____
7. _____
8. _____
9. _____
10. _____
11. _____
12. _____

13. _____

14. _____
15. _____
16. _____
17. _____
18. _____
19. _____
20. _____

21. _____
22. _____
23. _____

24. _____
25. _____

26. _____

27. _____
28. _____
29. _____
30. _____
31. _____
32. _____
33. _____
34. _____
35. _____

36. _____

37. _____

38. _____

39. _____
40. _____

41. _____

Figure 6.17

List of Structures, Deep Anterolateral View

Anterior scalene muscle
Axillary artery
Axillary vein
Buccinator muscle
Esophagus
External carotid artery
External jugular vein

Hyoid bone
Internal carotid artery
Internal jugular vein
Mastoid process
Middle scalene muscle
Posterior scalene muscle
Submandibular salivary gland

Sternocleidomastoid muscle
Styloid process
Thyrohyoid membrane
Thyroid cartilage
Thyroid gland
Trachea

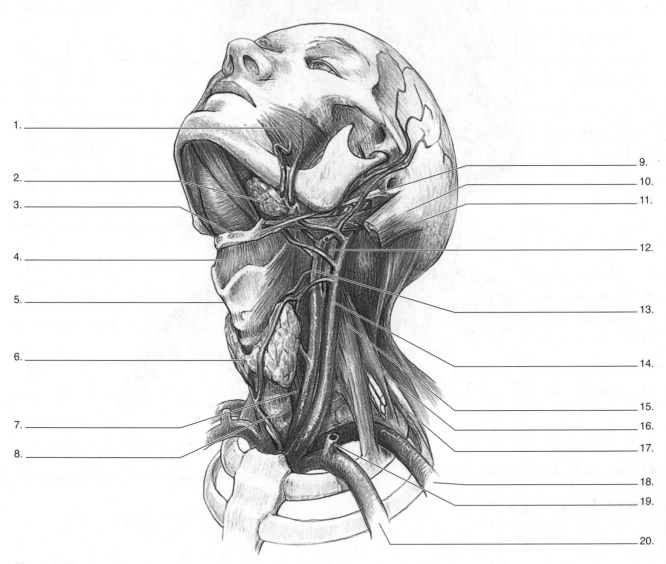

1.
2.
3.
4.
5.
6.
7.
8.
9.
10.
11.
12.
13.
14.
15.
16.
17.
18.
19.
20.

Figure 6.18

List of Structures, Cervical Vertebra Superior View

Annulus fibrosus
Anterior longitudinal ligament
Arachnoid mater
Dorsal root of spinal nerve
Dura mater
Internal vertebral venous plexus

Nucleus pulposus
Pia mater
Posterior longitudinal
  ligament
Spinal cord
Spinal nerve roots

Spinous process
Superior articular facet
Ventral root of spinal nerve
Vertebral artery
Vertebral body
Vertebral veins

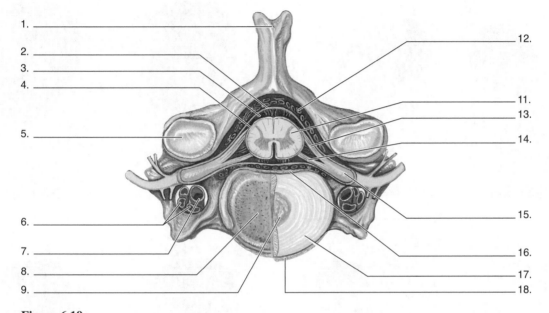

Figure 6.19

OUTLINE AND LABEL BORDERS OF CAUTION SITES

Recall from the text that the anterior and posterior triangles are sites of caution and contain a multitude of special structures.

INSTRUCTIONS. Outline and label the borders of the anterior and posterior triangles using the image below.

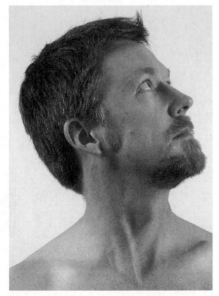

Figure 6.20

IDENTIFY NECK AND JAW MOVEMENTS

In this activity, you will identify the individual movements of the neck and jaw.

INSTRUCTIONS. Beneath each of the following figures, write the name of each movement.

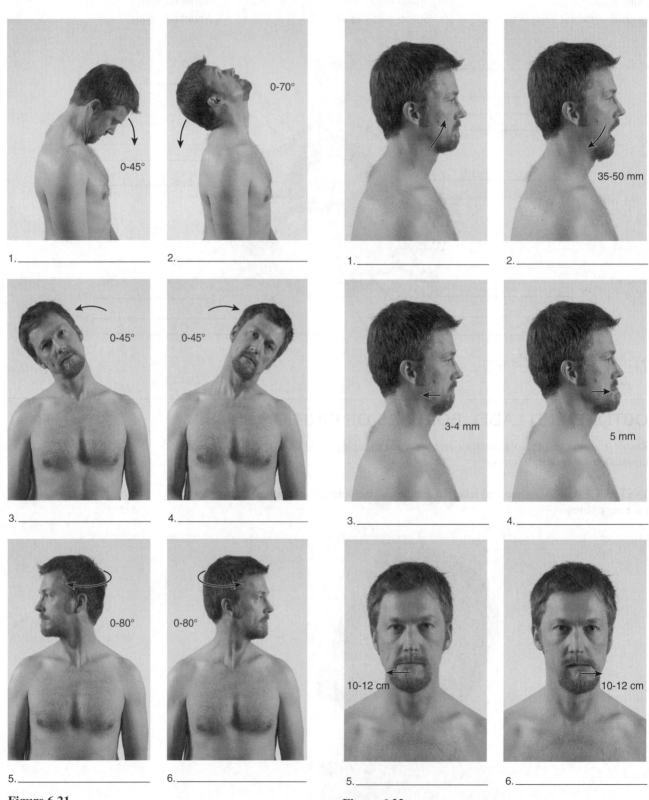

1._____   2._____

3._____   4._____

5._____   6._____

Figure 6.21

1._____   2._____

3._____   4._____

5._____   6._____

Figure 6.22

MATCH MUSCLE ORIGINS, INSERTIONS, AND ACTIONS

Each muscle has unique muscle attachments, crosses a specific joint or joints, and performs specific movements.

INSTRUCTIONS. Match each muscle of the head, neck, and face with the corresponding origin. Answers may be used more than once.

1. _____ Digastric
2. _____ Infrahyoids
3. _____ Lateral pterygoid
4. _____ Longus capitis
5. _____ Longus colli
6. _____ Masseter
7. _____ Medial pterygoid
8. _____ Obliquus capitis inferior
9. _____ Obliquus capitis superior
10. _____ Platysma
11. _____ Rectus capitis anterior
12. _____ Rectus capitis lateralis
13. _____ Rectus capitis posterior major
14. _____ Rectus capitis posterior minor
15. _____ Scalenes
16. _____ Semispinalis
17. _____ Splenius capitis
18. _____ Splenius cervicis
19. _____ Sternocleidomastoid
20. _____ Suprahyoids
21. _____ Temporalis

A. Transverse processes of C4–T10

B. Fascia of superior pectoralis major and deltoid muscles

C. Inferior border of mandible and mastoid process of temporal bone

D. Lateral pterygoid plate of sphenoid, palatine bone, and maxillary tuberosity

E. Lateral pterygoid plate, greater wing, and infratemporal crest of sphenoid

F. Ligamentum nuchae and spinous processes of C7–T3

G. Manubrium of sternum, thyroid cartilage, and superior border of scapula

H. Posterior arch of atlas (C1)

I. Spinous process of axis (C2)

J. Spinous processes of T3–T6

K. Superior manubrium of sternum and medial clavicle

L. Temporal fossa and fascia

M. Transverse process of atlas (C1)

N. Transverse processes of C2–C7

O. Transverse processes of C3–C5 and anterior bodies of C5–T3

P. Transverse processes of C3–C6

Q. Underside of mandible and styloid process of temporal bone

R. Zygomatic arch

INSTRUCTIONS. Match each muscle of the head, neck, and face with the corresponding insertion. Answers may be used more than once.

1. _____ Digastric
2. _____ Infrahyoids
3. _____ Lateral pterygoid
4. _____ Longus capitis
5. _____ Longus colli
6. _____ Masseter
7. _____ Medial pterygoid
8. _____ Obliquus capitis inferior
9. _____ Obliquus capitis superior
10. _____ Platysma
11. _____ Rectus capitis anterior
12. _____ Rectus capitis lateralis
13. _____ Rectus capitis posterior major
14. _____ Rectus capitis posterior minor
15. _____ Scalenes
16. _____ Semispinalis
17. _____ Splenius capitis
18. _____ Splenius cervicis
19. _____ Sternocleidomastoid
20. _____ Suprahyoids
21. _____ Temporalis

A. Angle, ramus, and coronoid process of mandible
B. Anterior surfaces of C2–C6
C. Between superior and inferior nuchal lines of occiput
D. Between superior and inferior nuchal lines of occiput and spinous processes of C2–T4
E. Condyle of mandible and articular disk
F. Coronoid process and anterior border of ramus of mandible
G. First and second ribs
H. Hyoid bone
I. Hyoid bone and thyroid cartilage
J. Inferior border of mandible
K. Inferior surface of basilar portion of occiput
L. Inferior surface of basilar portion of occiput
M. Mastoid process of temporal bone
N. Interior surface of angle and ramus of mandible
O. Lateral part of inferior nuchal line of occiput
P. Mastoid process and lateral portion of superior nuchal line of occiput
Q. Medial part of inferior nuchal line of occiput
R. Transverse process of atlas (C1)
S. Transverse processes of C1–C3

INSTRUCTIONS. Match each muscle of the head, neck, and face with the corresponding actions. Choose all that apply. Some answers will be used more than once.

1. _____ Digastric
2. _____ Lateral pterygoid
3. _____ Longus capitis
4. _____ Longus colli
5. _____ Masseter
6. _____ Medial pterygoid
7. _____ Obliquus capitis inferior
8. _____ Obliquus capitis superior
9. _____ Platysma
10. _____ Rectus capitis anterior
11. _____ Rectus capitis lateralis
12. _____ Rectus capitis posterior major
13. _____ Rectus capitis posterior minor
14. _____ Scalenes
15. _____ Semispinalis
16. _____ Splenius capitis
17. _____ Splenius cervicis
18. _____ Sternocleidomastoid
19. _____ Suprahyoids
20. _____ Temporalis

A. Depress mandible
B. Elevate mandible
C. Extend head and neck
D. Flex head and neck
E. Laterally deviate mandible
F. Laterally flex head and neck
G. Protract mandible
H. Retract mandible
I. Rotate head and neck to opposite side
J. Rotate head and neck to same side

IDENTIFY SHORTENING AND LENGTHENING MUSCLES

This activity will help you become more familiar with muscles of the head, neck, and face.

INSTRUCTIONS. For each of the following muscles, identify the position where the muscle is most shortened and the position that lengthens or stretches the muscle. (Hint: Moving into the muscle actions will shorten the muscle and reversing them will lengthen or stretch it.)

Longus Colli

Shortened position: _____

_____

Lengthened position: _____

_____

Masseter

Shortened position: _____

_____

Lengthened position: _____

_____

Scalenes

Shortened position: _____

_____

Lengthened position: _____

_____

Semispinalis

Shortened position: _____

_____

Lengthened position: _____

_____

Splenius Capitis

Shortened position: _____

_____

Lengthened position: _____

_____

Sternocleidomastoid

Shortened position: _____

_____

Lengthened position: _____

_____

Temporalis

Shortened position: _____

_____

Lengthened position: _____

_____

COMPLETE THE TABLE: SYNERGISTS/ANTAGONISTS

The next activity will help you gain a better sense of how the muscles of the head, neck, and face work together or in opposition.

INSTRUCTIONS. Fill in the missing information about muscles of the head, neck, and face. The first column indicates a movement of the neck or jaw, the second identifies which muscles perform this action, and the third indicates the opposite action. The first one is completed for you as an example.

Movement	Muscles	Opposite Action
Jaw depression	Suprahyoids Digastric Lateral pterygoid	Jaw elevation
Jaw elevation		
Jaw left lateral deviation		
Jaw protraction		
Jaw retraction		

(*Continued on next page*)

Movement	Muscles	Opposite Action
Jaw right lateral deviation		
Neck extension		
Neck flexion		
Neck left lateral flexion		
Neck left rotation		
Neck right lateral flexion		
Neck right rotation		

PUTTING THE HEAD, NECK, AND FACE IN MOTION

The following activity brings together all that you have learned about the head, neck, and face. As you examine several specific movements, describe: (1) which joints are involved, (2) which joint motions occur, and (3) in what sequence these occur. It is often helpful to perform the movement yourself, observe someone else performing the movement, or watch an animation or video of the movement to better understand what is happening and when.

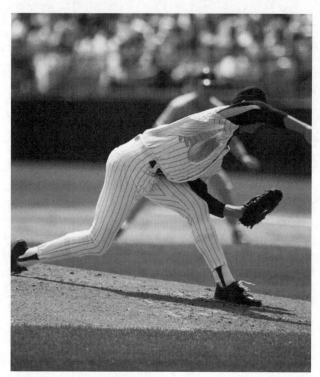

Figure 6.23 Overhand Throw

INSTRUCTIONS. List the joints involved in the movement shown.

_____

_____

_____

INSTRUCTIONS. List the motions that occur at each joint.

_____

_____

_____

INSTRUCTIONS. List the sequence of events involved in the movement shown.

_____

_____

_____

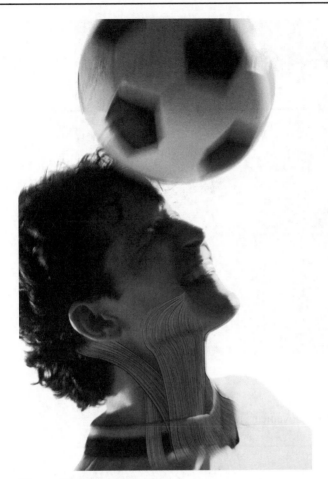

Figure 6.24 Soccer Header

INSTRUCTIONS. List the joints involved in the movement shown.

_____

_____

_____

INSTRUCTIONS. List the motions that occur at each joint.

_____

_____

_____

INSTRUCTIONS. List the sequence of events involved in the movement shown.

_____

_____

_____

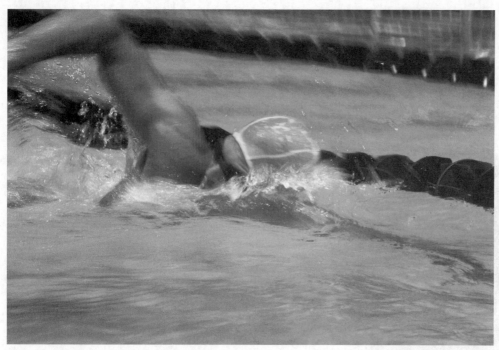

Figure 6.25 Swimming: Crawl Stroke

INSTRUCTIONS. List the joints involved in the movement shown.

_____

_____

_____

INSTRUCTIONS. List the motions that occur at each joint.

_____

_____

_____

INSTRUCTIONS. List the sequence of events involved in the movement shown.

_____

_____

_____

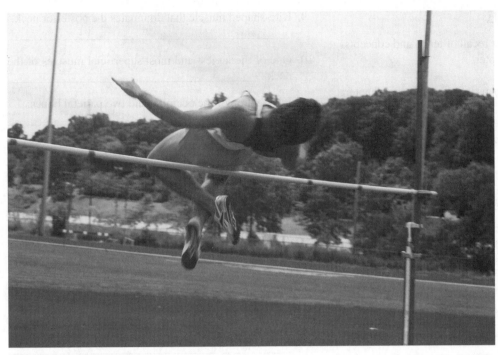

Figure 6.26 High Jump

INSTRUCTIONS. List the joints involved in the movement shown.

_____

_____

_____

INSTRUCTIONS. List the motions that occur at each joint.

_____

_____

_____

INSTRUCTIONS. List the sequence of events involved in the movement shown.

_____

_____

_____

WORD CHALLENGE

This final exercise checks your recall of terms and concepts introduced throughout the chapter.

INSTRUCTIONS. Twenty terms introduced in this chapter are hidden in the word search puzzle. Locate each term, and write it next to its numbered definition. Terms may be found horizontally, vertically, or diagonally.

List of Terms

1. Small, two-bellied muscle located under the mandible. _____

2. First cervical vertebra. _____

3. Second cervical vertebra. _____

4. Articulates with the mandible at the temporomandibular joint. _____

5. Intermediate muscle of neck. _____

6. Facial muscle that helps us smile. _____

7. Thick, strong muscle that extends between the zygomatic arch and the mandible. _____

8. Term for the most posterior part of the skull. _____

9. Kite-shaped muscle that dominates the posterior neck. _____

10. One of the largest and most superficial muscles of the neck. _____

11. Intersection of the occipital and two parietal bones. _____

12. The lower jaw bone. _____

13. Commonly called the "windpipe." _____

14. A "middle wing" that helps us chew. _____

15. Bony prominence of the temporal bone that articulates with the zygomatic bone. _____

16. Large bone of the central face. _____

17. Odontoid process. _____

18. Forms the medial wall of each orbit. _____

19. Commonly called the eye socket. _____

20. Adam's apple. _____

```
F Q U H M Q P B D P W I C K U D E N S J H V
Z O K R K R M P R K T B K L V C O Q L N W H
H P M R I O F T Q Z P Y M E Y E H G X R M X
X Q V W O Q B E N J N E T E R D D R A L D G
E E W Q C P X S K K M D G Y B A O O P Q Y H
Q X I K M E D I A L P T E R Y G O I D M H O
C N E R T N T Q H X A I B A Q X J L O V S Q
U Z Z M R E W W H V D C H S L E I N I X R K
U X Y Z O W F N B J I I R N M L B S Y X S I
R O D G E M V V N Q G Z O I O C I O H R T I
Y V V H O U C G C Y A P C Y M A O X Z L E M
M B B A E M W J M K S U C D H A G Q A L R U
A V I H L R A J N K T N I A S O L V D M N R
S S B Q W Q K T I K R G P N E N M B I K O I
S S S R U T X H I A I M U V P S O O O P C S
E E Z O R B I T H C C T T W A O Y W C N L O
T N G Q F F B T R A P E Z I U S C F B S E R
E R T H Y R O I D C A R T I L A G E Z A I I
R G A A C Z A U Q V G Z O Z B U C N V C D U
A T T C S X A L A M B D A C E S U O O T O S
K B L X H V S N U N A A N Q E U S X S K M N
O D A W I E I K F B I N E Z N S V E U A A F
E S S Q X U A V S W I J D M S E S V O Y S M
B G P N V M A I G R D D X I Y D Z J U Y T M
D L B L C S X R V B D C N P B O Z O G F O E
E Y R A F A E L N A I L P A D L P Z U C I P
U T Z B C J H E O O H U L Q M N E C B G D I
M G C A E K G V S O I C D A W I R F S T W F
```

Trunk

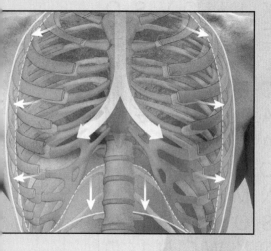

Our exploration of the axial skeleton continues in this segment with the trunk. Twelve thoracic vertebrae connect with 12 pairs of ribs, which curve around to join anteriorly with the costocartilage and flat sternum to form the rib cage. Five sturdy lumbar vertebrae form the base of the vertebral column, inferior to which are the sacrum and coccyx, which also form the posterior section of the pelvic girdle. The trunk houses many important internal organs and must offer solid protection without sacrificing mobility. Muscles and ligaments work together to produce movement and maintain balanced, upright posture over the lower extremities.

LABEL SURFACE LANDMARKS

The following activities will help familiarize you with the spine, ribs, sacrum, and ilium posteriorly and the chest, ribs, abdomen, and pelvis anteriorly.

INSTRUCTIONS. The following images depict the major surface landmarks of the trunk. Label each of the following in the spaces provided.

List of Structures, Anterior View

Iliac crest
Inguinal ligament
Linea alba

Pectoralis major
Rectus abdominis
Sternum

Umbilicus
Xiphoid process of sternum

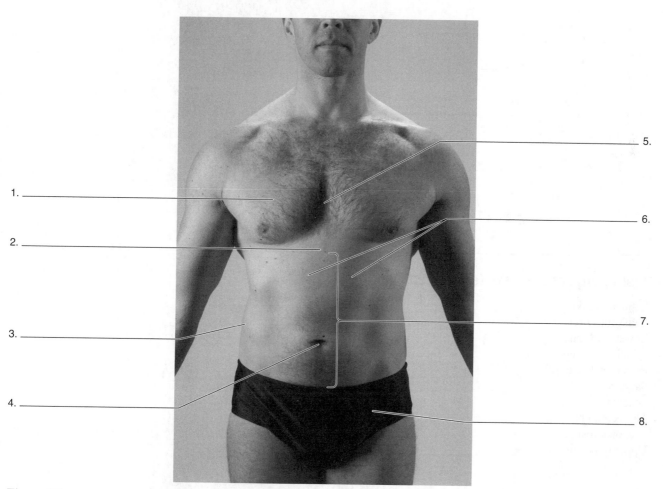

Figure 7.1

List of Structures, Anterolateral View

Anterior superior iliac spine
External oblique
Iliac crest
Pectoralis major
Rectus abdominis

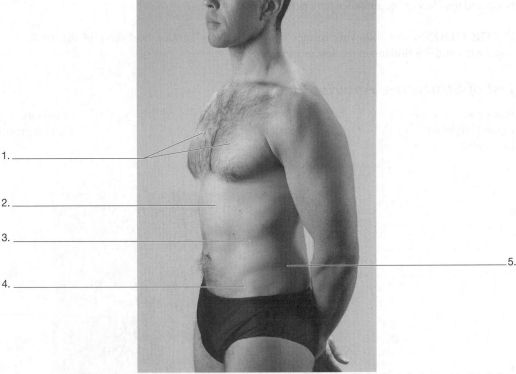

Figure 7.2

List of Structures, Posterior View

Lamina groove
Latissimus dorsi
Lower trapezius
Middle trapezius
Posterior iliac crest
Sacrum
Scapula
Thoracolumbar
 aponeurosis
Upper trapezius

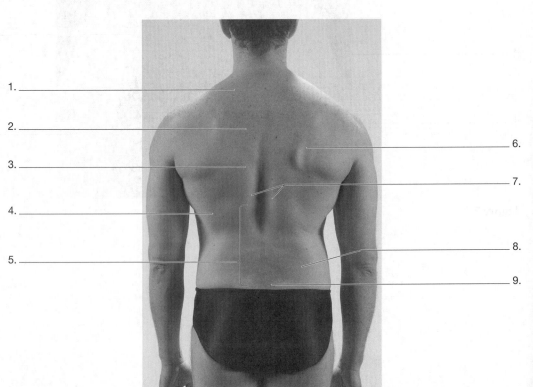

Figure 7.3

COLOR AND LABEL SKELETAL STRUCTURES

Bones and bony landmarks provide consistent touchstones as we locate, differentiate, and explore soft-tissue structures such as muscles, tendons, and ligaments.

INSTRUCTIONS. The following images depict the bones and bony landmarks for the trunk. Color and label each of the following structures.

List of Structures, Posterior View

Coccyx	Ischium	Scapula
Costovertebral joints	Pubis	Spinous processes
False ribs	Sacroiliac joints	Transverse processes
Floating ribs	Sacrum	True ribs
Ilium		

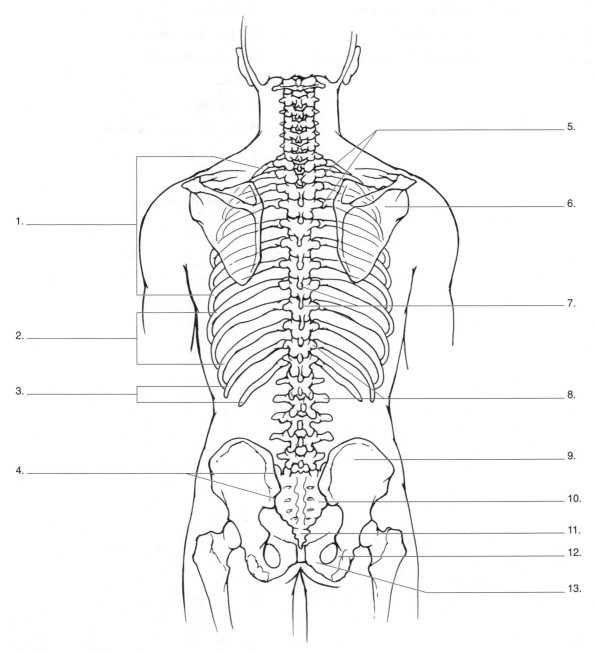

Figure 7.4

INSTRUCTIONS. Match each of the following bony landmarks with the corresponding muscle or muscles of the trunk. Choose all that apply. Some answers will be used more than once.

1. _____ Anterior ribs

2. _____ Costal cartilage

3. _____ Iliac crest

4. _____ Mastoid process

5. _____ Occiput

6. _____ Posterior ribs

7. _____ Posterior sacrum

8. _____ Posterior superior iliac spine

9. _____ Spinous processes

10. _____ Transverse processes

11. _____ Twelfth rib

12. _____ Xiphoid process of sternum

A. Diaphragm

B. External intercostals

C. External oblique

D. Iliocostalis

E. Internal intercostals

F. Internal oblique

G. Interspinalis

H. Intertransversarii

I. Longissimus

J. Multifidi

K. Quadratus lumborum

L. Rectus abdominis

M. Rotatores

N. Semispinalis

O. Serratus posterior inferior

P. Serratus posterior superior

Q. Spinalis

R. Transverse abdominis

LABEL JOINTS AND LIGAMENTS

The trunk relies on the small, gliding motions of individual vertebral facet joints for its mobility. Collectively, these joints are capable of relatively large movements in all three planes. The breathing mechanism is also driven by muscles in the trunk and requires mobility in the rib cage. These labeling activities help you explore the joints of the trunk and the ligaments that hold them together.

INSTRUCTIONS. The following images depict the bones and ligaments of the trunk. Label the structures listed.

List of Structures, Curvatures of the Spinal Column Lateral View

Atlas	Cervical curvature	Sacral curvature
Axis	Lumbar curvature	Thoracic curvature

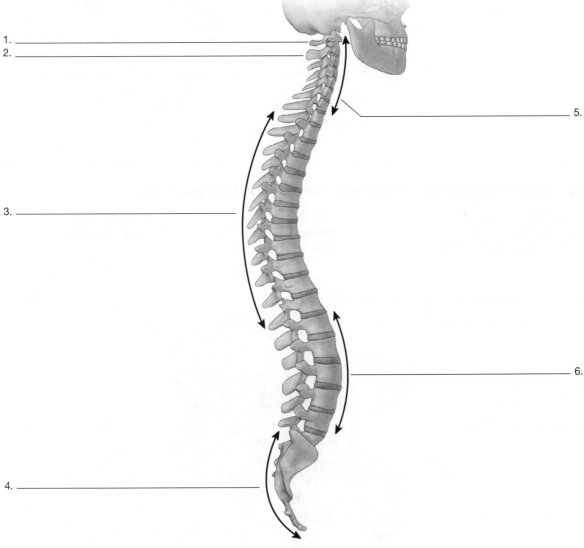

1. _____
2. _____

3. _____

4. _____

5. _____

6. _____

Figure 7.5

List of Structures, Thoracic Vertebra Posterolateral Oblique View

Costal facet of transverse process
Inferior costal facet
Lamina
Spinous process
Superior articular facet
Superior costal facet
Transverse process
Vertebral body

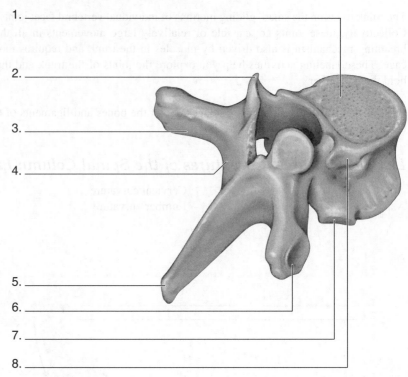

1. _____

2. _____

3. _____

4. _____

5. _____

6. _____

7. _____

8. _____

Figure 7.6

List of Structures, Lumbar Vertebra Posterolateral Oblique View

Articular facet of the superior
    articular process
Facet of the inferior articular process

Lamina
Spinous process
Transverse process

Vertebral body
Vertebral foramen

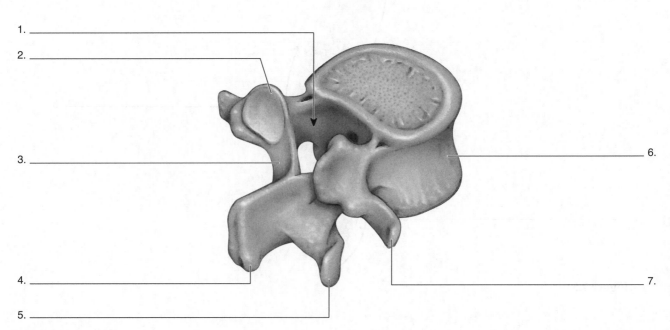

1. _____

2. _____

3. _____

4. _____

5. _____

6. _____

7. _____

Figure 7.7

List of Structures, Sacrum Anterior View

Ala
Anterior sacral foramina
Apex
Coccygeal vertebrae

Coccyx
Lumbosacral articular surface
Sacral promontory
Superior articular process

Transverse process of first coccygeal
    vertebra
Transverse ridges

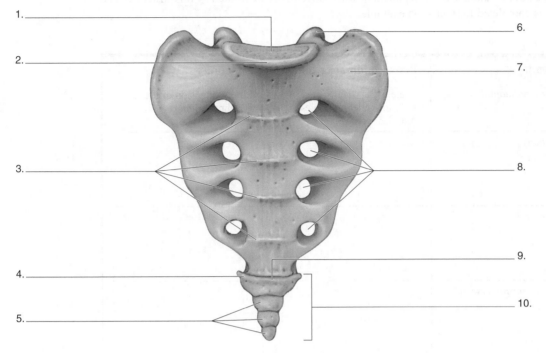

Figure 7.8

List of Structures, Sacrum Posterior View

Ala
Coccygeal cornu
Facet of superior
    articular process
Intermediate and
    lateral sacral crests
Median sacral crest
Posterior sacral
    foramina
Sacral canal
Sacral cornu
Sacral hiatus
Sacrospinous
    tubercles

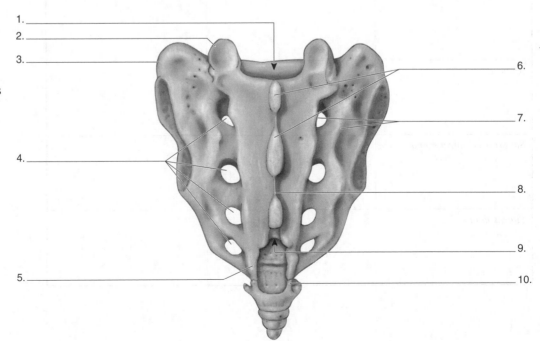

Figure 7.9

COMPLETE THE TABLE: LIGAMENTS

This activity will help you review the functions of the various ligaments.

INSTRUCTIONS. Fill in the missing information about ligaments of the trunk. The first column indicates a ligament of this region, the second identifies which bony landmarks it joins, and the third indicates the function of the ligament or what movements are limited by this structure. The first one is completed for you as an example.

Ligament	Bony Landmarks Joined	Function
Anterior longitudinal	Occiput Anterior vertebral bodies Anterior sacrum	Limits extension of the vertebral column
Interspinous		
Intertransverse		
Lateral costotransverse		
Ligamentum flavum		
Posterior longitudinal		
Radiate		
Superior costotransverse		
Supraspinous		

LABEL MUSCLES OF THE TRUNK

Several layers of muscles are necessary to move the trunk, maintain posture and alignment, draw breath in and force it out, and protect underlying structures. Broad, superficial muscles cover the chest, abdomen, and back while more intricate groups of muscles position the vertebral column and regulate breath.

INSTRUCTIONS. The following diagrams depict the superficial muscles of the trunk. Label each of the following structures:

List of Structures, Anterior View

Abdominal fascia
Deltoid
External oblique
Latissimus dorsi
Pectoralis major
Serratus anterior
Sternocleidomastoid

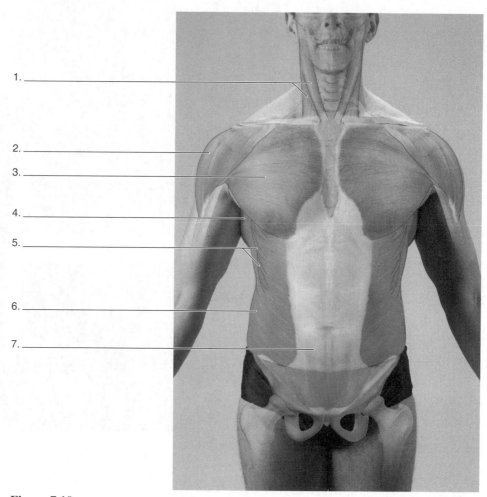

1. _____
2. _____
3. _____
4. _____
5. _____
6. _____
7. _____

Figure 7.10

List of Structures, Posterior View

Latissimus dorsi
Trapezius

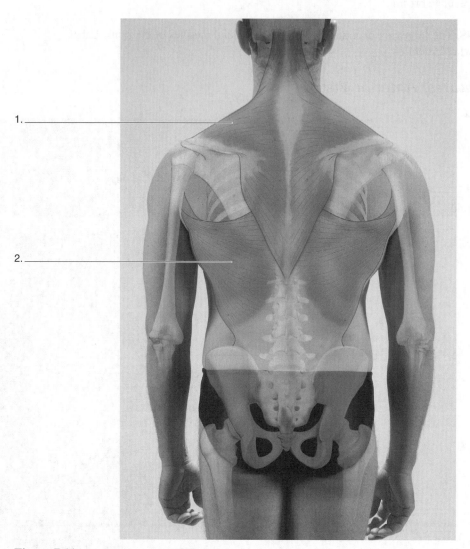

1.

2.

Figure 7.11

INSTRUCTIONS. The following diagrams depict the intermediate muscles of the trunk. Label each of the following structures.

List of Structures, Anterior View

Abdominal fascia
Intercostals
Internal obliques
Serratus anterior

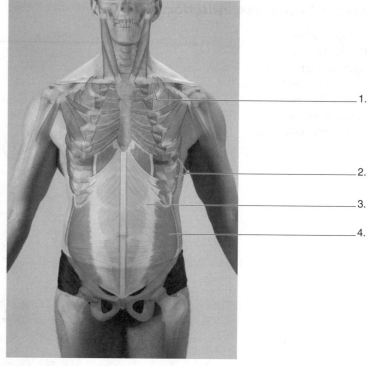

Figure 7.12

1. _____
2. _____
3. _____
4. _____

List of Structures, Posterior View

External oblique
Iliocostalis
Intercostals
Longissimus (use twice)
Rhomboid major
Rhomboid minor
Spinalis
Thoracolumbar aponeurosis

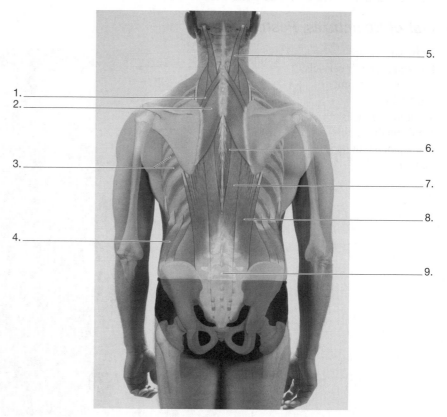

1. _____
2. _____
3. _____
4. _____
5. _____
6. _____
7. _____
8. _____
9. _____

Figure 7.13

INSTRUCTIONS. The following diagrams depict the deep muscles of the trunk. Label each of the following structures.

List of Structures, Anterior View

Coracobrachialis
External intercostals
Internal intercostals
Pectoralis minor
Rectus abdominis
Serratus anterior
Transverse abdominis

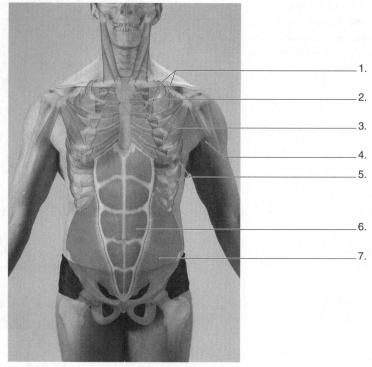

Figure 7.14

List of Structures, Posterior View

Intertransversarii
Intertransversarii cervicis
Levatores costarum
Multifidus
Rotatores thoracis
Semispinalis capitis
Semispinalis thoracis
Tendon

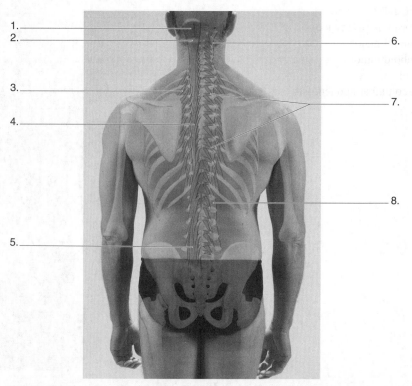

Figure 7.15

INSTRUCTIONS. The following diagrams depict the muscles of breathing. Label each of the following structures:

List of Structures, Anterior View

Diaphragm
External intercostals
External oblique
Internal intercostals

Internal oblique
Rectus abdominis
Scalenes

Serratus anterior
Sternocleidomastoid
Transverse thoracis

1. _____
2. _____
3. _____
4. _____
5. _____
6. _____

7. _____
8. _____
9. _____
10. _____

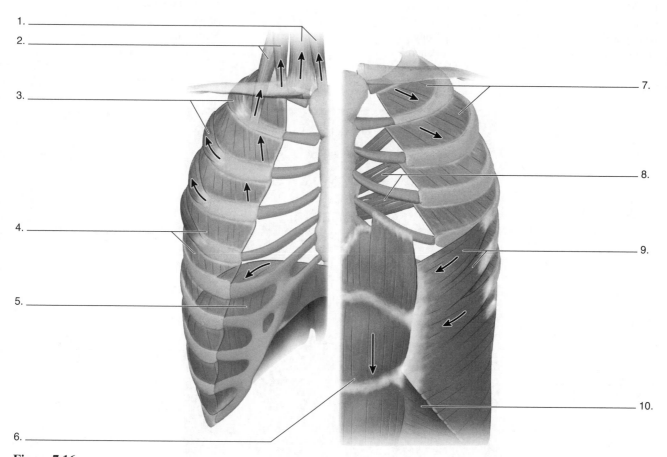

Figure 7.16

LABEL SPECIAL STRUCTURES

Several important structures are located in the trunk in addition to those directly responsible for movement. We must be aware of abdominal organs, blood vessels, lymph nodes and vessels, and nerves when palpating and working in this area.

INSTRUCTIONS. Label each of the following special structures of the head, neck, and face.

List of Structures, Anterior View of Viscera

Bladder	Heart	Small intestine
Colon	Liver	Spleen
Diaphragm	Lungs	Stomach
Gallbladder	Pancreas	

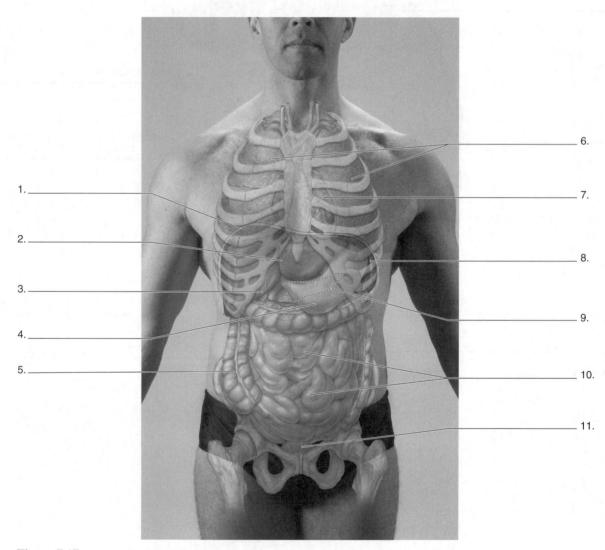

1. _____
2. _____
3. _____
4. _____
5. _____

6. _____
7. _____
8. _____
9. _____
10. _____
11. _____

Figure 7.17

List of Structures, Posterior View of Viscera

Appendix
Ascending colon
Bladder
Descending colon
Diaphragm (left dome)

Left kidney
Liver
Pancreas (outline)
Right adrenal gland

Right kidney
Right lung
Small intestine
Spleen

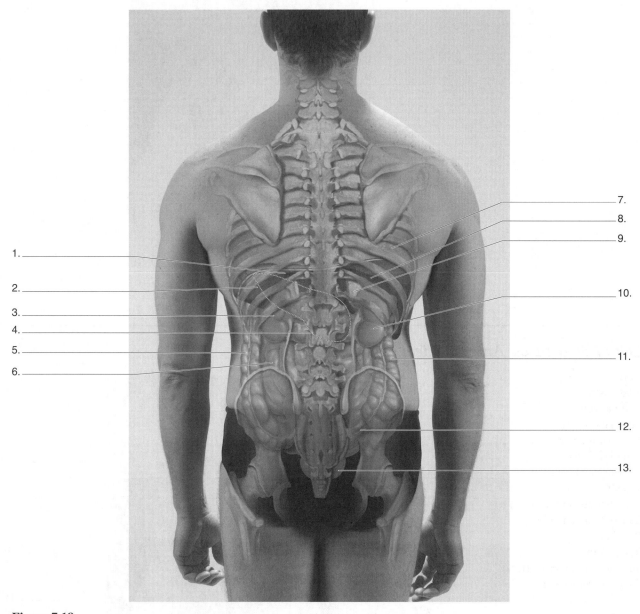

1.

2.

3.

4.

5.

6.

7.

8.

9.

10.

11.

12.

13.

Figure 7.18

List of Structures, Anterior View of Lymphatics

Cisterna chyli
Right lymphatic duct
Thoracic duct
Left internal jugular vein
Left subclavian vein

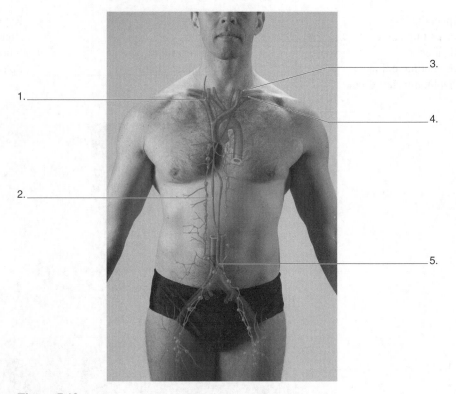

Figure 7.19

List of Structures, Anterior View of Blood Vessels

Aorta
Aortic arch
Cardiac vein
Coronary artery
External iliac arteries
Femoral veins
Inferior vena cava
Kidney
Left subclavian artery
Left subclavian vein
Renal artery
Renal vein
Superior mesenteric artery
Superior vena cava

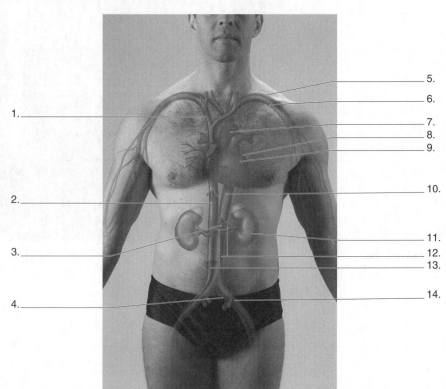

Figure 7.20

List of Structures, Anterior View of Nerves

Hepatic plexus
Inferior gluteal nerve
Lumbar plexus

Sacral plexus
Sciatic nerve

Splanchnic nerves
Superior gluteal nerve

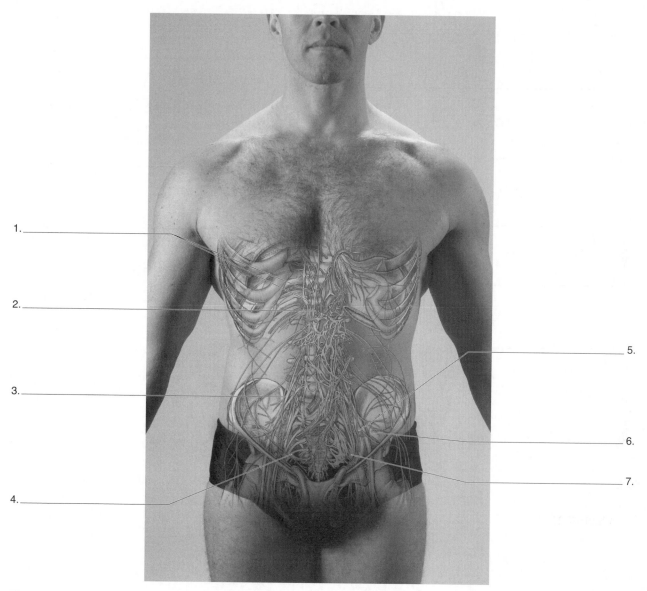

1.

2.

3.

4.

5.

6.

7.

Figure 7.21

List of Structures, Posterior View of Nerves

C8 spinal nerve
Cauda equina
Cervical enlargement of spinal cord
External intercostal muscle

First cervical spinal nerve
First lumbar spinal nerve
Intercostal nerves
Lumbar enlargement of spinal cord

Pedicle of cervical vertebra
Psoas major muscle
T5 spinal nerve
Transverse abdominal muscle

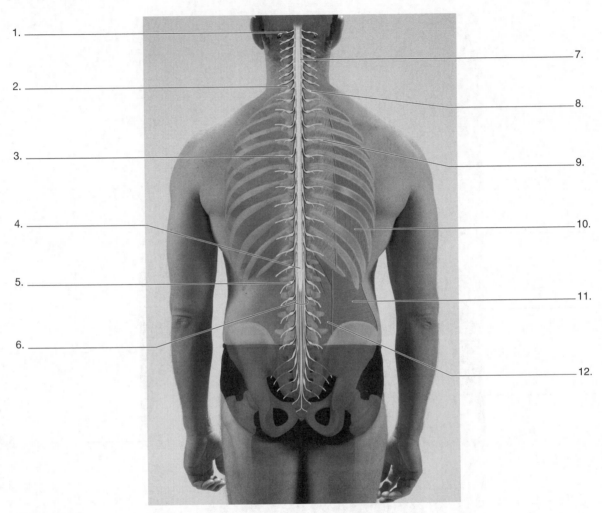

1. ———
2. ———
3. ———
4. ———
5. ———
6. ———

7. ———
8. ———
9. ———
10. ———
11. ———
12. ———

Figure 7.22

IDENTIFY TRUNK MOVEMENTS

Movements in the trunk position the entire upper body, extend the range of the extremities, and transfer forces between different body regions. The mobility of this region directly affects the ease and depth of breathing. This activity will help you study movements of the trunk, including movements of breathing.

INSTRUCTIONS. Beneath each of the following figures, write the name of each movement.

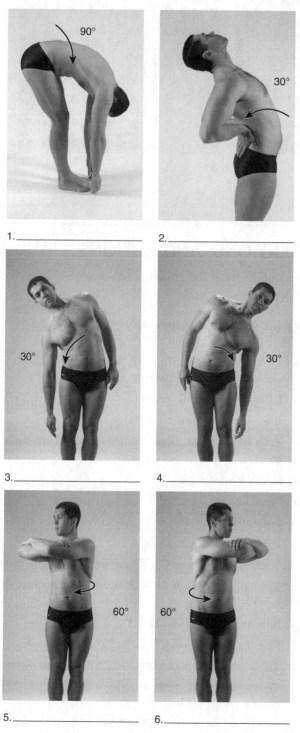

1._____   2._____

3._____   4._____

5._____   6._____

Figure 7.23

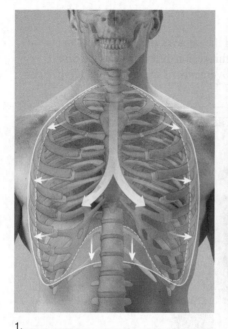 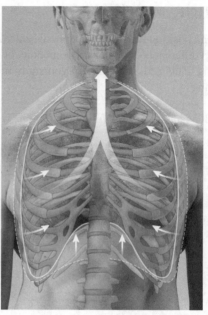

1._____   2._____

Figure 7.24

MATCH MUSCLE ORIGINS, INSERTIONS, AND ACTIONS

Now that we are more familiar with the structures of the trunk and groups of muscles, let's examine the individual muscles located in this region.

INSTRUCTIONS. Match each muscle of the trunk with the corresponding origin. Some answers may be used more than once.

1. _____ Diaphragm

2. _____ External intercostals

3. _____ External oblique

4. _____ Iliocostalis

5. _____ Internal intercostals

6. _____ Internal oblique

7. _____ Interspinalis

8. _____ Intertransversarii

9. _____ Longissimus

10. _____ Multifidi

11. _____ Quadratus lumborum

12. _____ Rectus abdominis

13. _____ Rotatores

14. _____ Semispinalis

15. _____ Serratus posterior inferior

16. _____ Serratus posterior superior

17. _____ Spinalis

18. _____ Transverse abdominis

A. Costal cartilages of ribs 7–12, thoracolumbar fascia, internal iliac crest, and lateral inguinal ligament

B. External surfaces of ribs 5–12

C. Inner surface and costal cartilage of ribs

D. Inner surfaces and costal cartilages of ribs 7–12, xiphoid process, bodies of L1–L2 vertebrae

E. Lower border of rib

F. Posterior iliac crest and iliolumbar ligament

G. Posterior sacrum, medial lip of ilium, posterior surface of ribs 1–12

H. Pubic crest and symphysis

I. Spinous processes of C7–T3 and the ligamentum nuchae

J. Spinous processes of T11–L2, ligamentum nuchae, spinous processes C7–T2

K. Spinous processes of T11–L3

L. Spinous processes of C3–T2 and T12–L5

M. Thoracolumbar aponeurosis, iliac crest, lateral inguinal ligament

N. Thoracolumbar aponeurosis, transverse processes of T1–L5, articular processes of C4–C7

O. Transverse processes of C4–T12

P. Transverse processes of C1–L5

Q. Transverse processes of C4–L5, posterior sacrum, and posterior iliac spine

INSTRUCTIONS. Match each muscle of the trunk with the corresponding insertion. Some
answers may be used more than once.

1. _____ Diaphragm

2. _____ External intercostals

3. _____ External oblique

4. _____ Iliocostalis

5. _____ Internal intercostals

6. _____ Internal oblique

7. _____ Interspinalis

8. _____ Intertransversarii

9. _____ Longissimus

10. _____ Multifidi

11. _____ Quadratus lumborum

12. _____ Rectus abdominis

13. _____ Rotatores

14. _____ Semispinalis

15. _____ Serratus posterior inferior

16. _____ Serratus posterior superior

17. _____ Spinalis

18. _____ Transverse abdominis

A. Abdominal aponeurosis, crest and pectineal line of pubis

B. Abdominal aponeurosis, inguinal ligament, anterior crest of ilium

C. Abdominal aponeurosis and internal surfaces of ribs 10–12

D. Central tendon

E. Costal cartilage of ribs 5–7 and xiphoid process of sternum

F. Lower border of rib above

G. Posterior surfaces of ribs 2–5

H. Posterior surfaces of ribs 9–12

I. Spinous process 2–4 vertebra above in C2–L5

J. Spinous process of vertebra above

K. Spinous processes of C2–C4 and T1–T8 and between superior and inferior nuchal lines of occiput

L. Spinous processes of C2–T4 and occiput between superior and inferior nuchal lines

M. Transverse process of vertebra above

N. Transverse processes of C2–C6 and T1–T12, posterior surface of ribs 3–12, mastoid process

O. Transverse processes of C4–C7 and posterior surface of ribs 1–12

P. Transverse processes of L1–L4 and inferior border of 12th rib

INSTRUCTIONS. Match each muscle of the trunk with the corresponding actions. Answers
may be used more than once. Some items will have more than one correct answer.

1. _____ Diaphragm

2. _____ External intercostals

3. _____ External oblique

4. _____ Iliocostalis

5. _____ Internal intercostals

6. _____ Internal oblique

7. _____ Interspinalis

8. _____ Intertransversarii

9. _____ Longissimus

10. _____ Multifidi

11. _____ Quadratus lumborum

12. _____ Rectus abdominis

13. _____ Rotatores

14. _____ Semispinalis

15. _____ Serratus posterior inferior

16. _____ Serratus posterior superior

17. _____ Spinalis

18. _____ Transverse abdominis

A. Exhalation

B. Extend trunk

C. Flex trunk

D. Inhalation

E. Laterally flex trunk

F. Rotate trunk to opposite side

G. Rotate trunk to same side

IDENTIFY SHORTENING AND LENGTHENING TRUNK MUSCLES

This activity will help you become more familiar with each muscle of the trunk.

INSTRUCTIONS. For each of the following muscles, identify the position where the muscle is most shortened and the position that lengthens or stretches the muscle.

Erector Spinae Group

Shortened position: _____

_____

Lengthened position: _____

_____

External Oblique

Shortened position: _____

_____

Lengthened position: _____

_____

Internal Oblique

Shortened position: _____

_____

Lengthened position: _____

_____

Quadratus Lumborum

Shortened position: _____

_____

Lengthened position: _____

_____

Rectus Abdominis

Shortened position: _____

_____

Lengthened position: _____

_____

Semispinalis

Shortened position: _____

_____

Lengthened position: _____

_____

COMPLETE THE TABLE: SYNERGISTS/ANTAGONISTS

The following activity will help you gain a better sense of how the trunk muscles work together or in opposition.

INSTRUCTIONS. Fill in the missing information about muscles of the trunk. The first column indicates a movement, the second identifies which muscles perform this action, and the third indicates the opposite action. The first one is completed for you as an example.

Movement	Muscles	Opposite Action
Exhalation	External oblique Internal intercostals Internal oblique Rectus abdominis Serratus posterior inferior Subcostales Transverse abdominis Transversus thoracis	Inhalation
Inhalation		

(Continued on next page)

Movement	Muscles	Opposite Action
Trunk extension		
Trunk flexion		
Trunk left lateral flexion		
Trunk left rotation		
Trunk right lateral flexion		
Trunk right rotation		

PUTTING THE TRUNK IN MOTION

The following activity brings together all you have learned about the trunk. As in previous chapters, for each movement shown, you will describe: (1) the joints involved, (2) the joint motions that occur, and (3) in the sequence in which they occur. It is often helpful to perform the movement yourself, observe someone else performing the movement, or watch an animation or video of the movement to better understand what is happening and when.

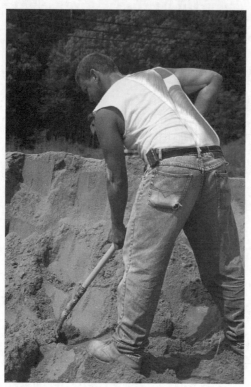

Figure 7.25 Shoveling

INSTRUCTIONS. List the joints involved in the movement shown.

_____

_____

_____

INSTRUCTIONS. List the motions that occur at each joint.

_____

_____

_____

INSTRUCTIONS. List the sequence of events involved in the movement shown.

_____

_____

_____

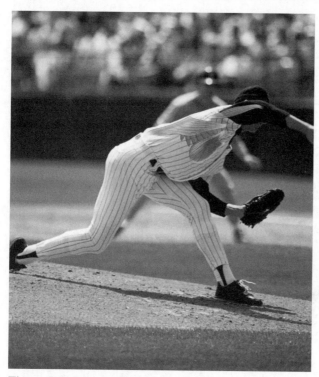

Figure 7.26 Overhand Throw

INSTRUCTIONS. List the joints involved in the movement shown.

_____

_____

_____

INSTRUCTIONS. List the motions that occur at each joint.

_____

_____

_____

INSTRUCTIONS. List the sequence of events involved in the movement shown.

_____

_____

_____

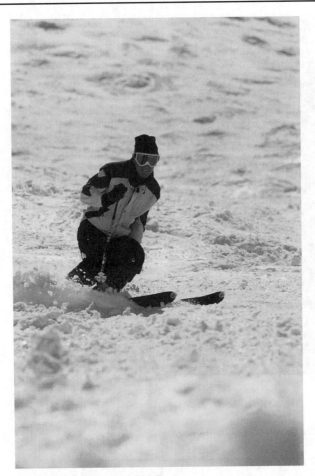

Figure 7.27 Downhill Ski Turn

INSTRUCTIONS. List the joints involved in the movement shown.

_____

_____

_____

INSTRUCTIONS. List the motions that occur at each joint.

_____

_____

_____

INSTRUCTIONS. List the sequence of events involved in the movement shown.

_____

_____

_____

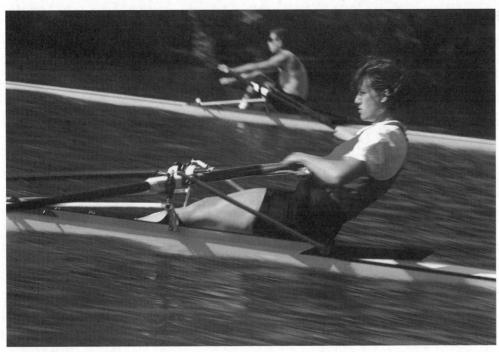

Figure 7.28 Rowing

INSTRUCTIONS. List the joints involved in the movement shown.

_____

_____

_____

INSTRUCTIONS. List the motions that occur at each joint.

_____

_____

_____

INSTRUCTIONS. List the sequence of events involved in the movement shown.

_____

_____

_____

WORD CHALLENGE

This final exercise checks your recall of terms and concepts introduced throughout the chapter.

INSTRUCTIONS. Unscramble each word and match it to its description.

1. licoisitoals _____

2. yesdink _____

3. deepcli _____

4. theapci lsepxu _____

5. tleevw _____

6. nonhaialti _____

7. drau tream _____

8. coolsisis _____

9. maidgraph _____

10. udaca uqenia _____

A. Group of nerves innervating the liver

B. Paired organs only partially protected by the inferior rib cage

C. Number of thoracic vertebrae

D. Most superficial of three meninges

E. Primary muscle of breathing

F. Most lateral of erector spinae muscles

G. Short "foot" projecting from vertebral body

H. The name means "horse's tail"

I. Pathologic lateral curvature of the spine

J. Movement in which expansion of the rib cage decreases air pressure within the thoracic cavity

Pelvis, Thigh, and Knee

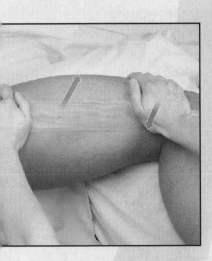

It is time to travel distally, to the lower extremity. The hip and knee work together to support or propel the body; therefore, stability and structural alignment are necessary. In addition, the hip and knee must lock into a single unit over the foot when supporting heavy loads and unlock into separate segments for variable positioning and movement. The following activities will help you understand the structure and function of the pelvis, thigh, and knee.

LABEL SURFACE LANDMARKS

This activity will help you familiarize yourself with surface landmarks and their relation to underlying structures.

INSTRUCTIONS. The following images depict the major surface landmarks of the lower extremity. Label each of the following in the spaces provided.

List of Structures, Anterior View

Femoral triangle	Patellar tendon	Vastus lateralis muscle
Iliac crest	Rectus femoris muscle	Vastus medialis muscle
Patella	Tensor fascia latae muscle	

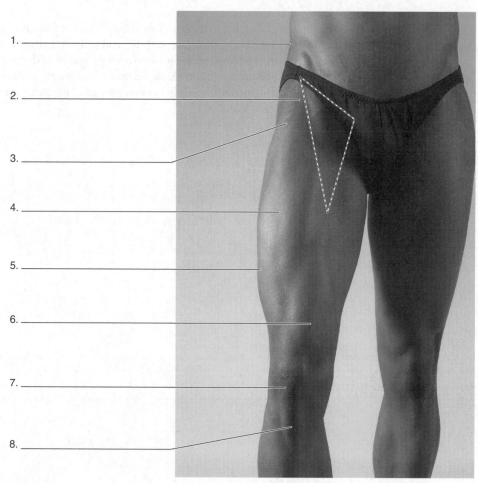

1. _____

2. _____

3. _____

4. _____

5. _____

6. _____

7. _____

8. _____

Figure 8.1

List of Structures, Lateral View

Biceps femoris muscle
Fibular head
Gluteus maximus muscle
Gluteus medius muscle
Greater trochanter
   of the femur
Iliac crest
Iliotibial band
Patella
Rectus femoris
   muscle
Tensor fascia
   latae muscle
Tibial tuberosity
Vastus lateralis
   muscle

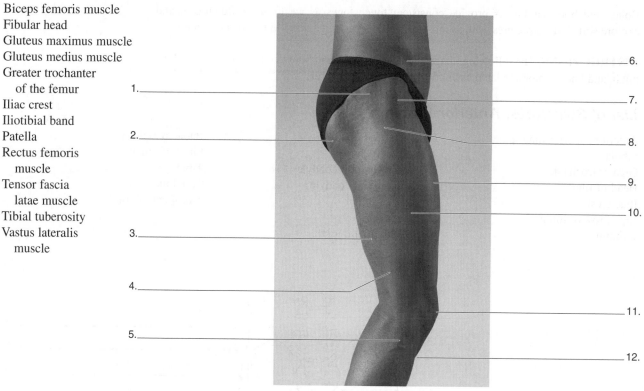

Figure 8.2

List of Structures, Posterior View

Adductor magnus muscle
Biceps femoris muscle
Gluteal fold
Gluteus maximus muscle
Gluteus medius muscle
Gracilis muscle
Pes anserine
   tendon
Popliteal fossa
Semimembranosus
   muscle
Semitendinosus
   muscle

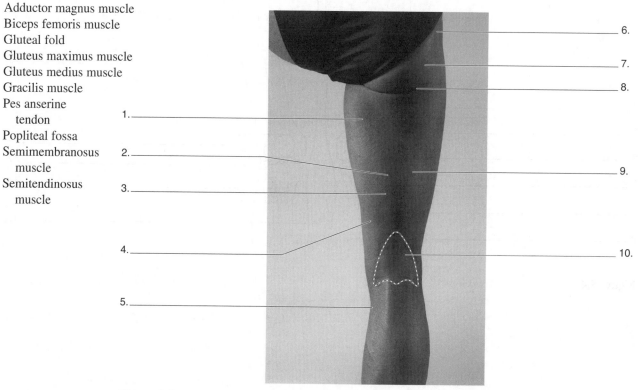

Figure 8.3

COLOR AND LABEL SKELETAL STRUCTURES

Bones and bony landmarks provide consistent touchstones as we locate, differentiate, and explore soft-tissue structures such as muscles, tendons, and ligaments in the lower extremity.

INSTRUCTIONS. The following images depict the bones and bony landmarks for the pelvis, thigh, and knee. Color and label each of the following structures.

List of Structures, Anterior View

Anterior superior iliac spine
Fibula
Greater trochanter
Head of fibula
Iliac crest
Iliac fossa of ilium
Ischium

Lateral femoral condyle
Lesser trochanter
Medial femoral condyle
Medial tibial condyle
Neck of femur
Patella
Patellofemoral joint

Pubic symphysis
Shaft of femur
Tibia
Tibial tuberosity
Tibiofemoral joint

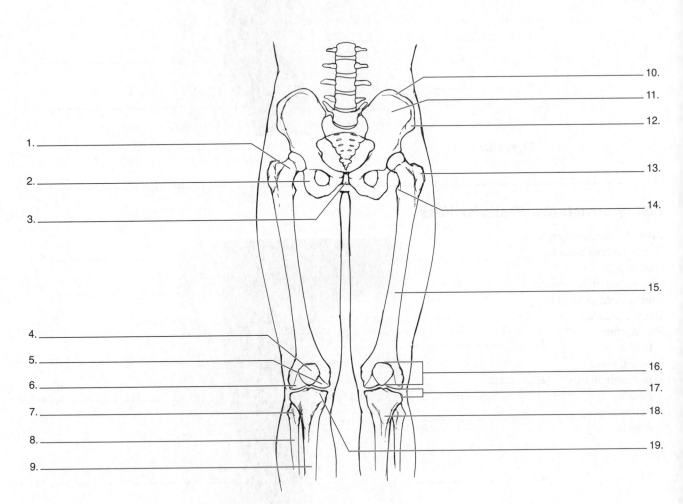

Figure 8.4

List of Structures, Posterior View

Coccyx
Femoral head
Femoral neck
Fibular head
Fifth lumbar vertebra (L5)
Greater trochanter
Ilium

Intercondylar notch
Ischial tuberosity
Lateral femoral condyle
Lateral tibial condyle
Lesser trochanter
Medial femoral condyle
Medial tibial condyle

Pectineal line
Posterior inferior iliac spine
Posterior superior iliac spine
Sacroiliac joint
Sacrum
Shaft of femur

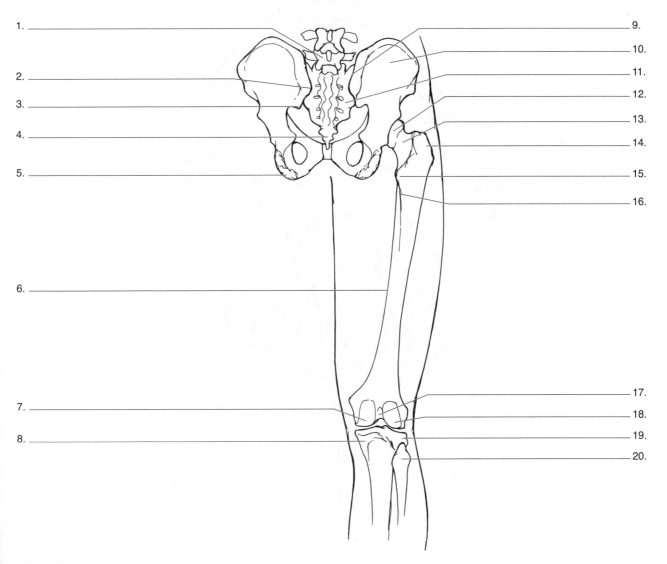

1. _____
2. _____
3. _____
4. _____
5. _____
6. _____
7. _____
8. _____

9. _____
10. _____
11. _____
12. _____
13. _____
14. _____
15. _____
16. _____
17. _____
18. _____
19. _____
20. _____

Figure 8.5

List of Structures, Pelvis Lateral View

Acetabulum
Anterior inferior iliac spine
Anterior superior iliac spine
Coccyx
Femoral head
Femoral shaft

Greater sciatic notch
Greater trochanter
Iliac crest
Inferior ramus of pubis
Ischial spine
Ischial tuberosity

Lesser sciatic notch
Posterior inferior iliac spine
Posterior superior iliac spine
Pubic tubercle
Sacrum
Superior ramus of pubis

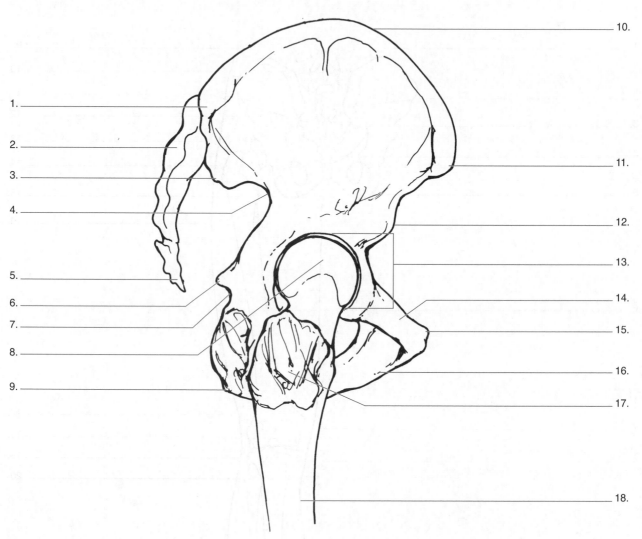

Figure 8.6

INSTRUCTIONS. Match each of the following bony landmarks with the corresponding muscle attachment. Choose all that apply. Answers may be used more than once.

1. _____ Adductor tubercle

2. _____ Anterior inferior iliac spine

3. _____ Anterior superior iliac spine

4. _____ Fibular head

5. _____ Greater trochanter

6. _____ Iliac fossa

7. _____ Ischium

8. _____ Lateral femoral condyle

9. _____ Lateral tibial condyle

10. _____ Lesser trochanter

11. _____ Medial femoral condyle

12. _____ Medial tibial condyle

13. _____ Posterior superior iliac spine

14. _____ Pubic rami

15. _____ Sacrum

16. _____ Tibial tuberosity

A. Psoas

B. Iliacus

C. Sartorius

D. Tensor fascia latae

E Quadriceps group

F. Adductor group

G. Gluteal group

H. Deep six lateral rotators

I. Hamstring group

J. Popliteus

LABEL JOINTS AND LIGAMENTS

This next activity will help you explore the joints of the pelvis, hip, and knee and the ligaments that hold them together.

INSTRUCTIONS. Label the following bones and ligaments of the pelvis, thigh, and knee.

List of Structures, Pelvis Posterior View

Iliofemoral ligament

Ischiofemoral ligament

Posterior sacrococcygeal ligament

Posterior sacroiliac ligaments

Sacrospinous ligament

Sacrotuberous ligament

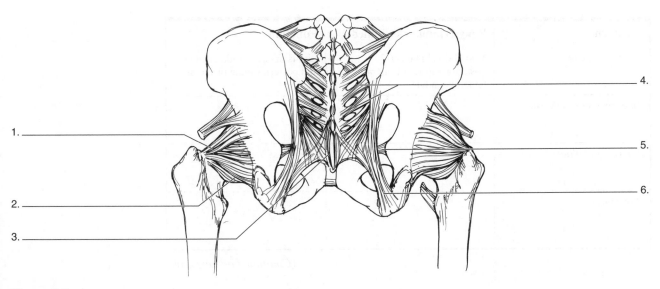

Figure 8.7

List of Structures, Knee Posterior View

Anterior cruciate ligament
Femur
Fibula
Lateral collateral ligament

Lateral meniscus
Medial collateral ligament
Medial meniscus
Posterior cruciate ligament

Posterior meniscofemoral
  ligament
Proximal tibiofibular joint capsule
Tibia

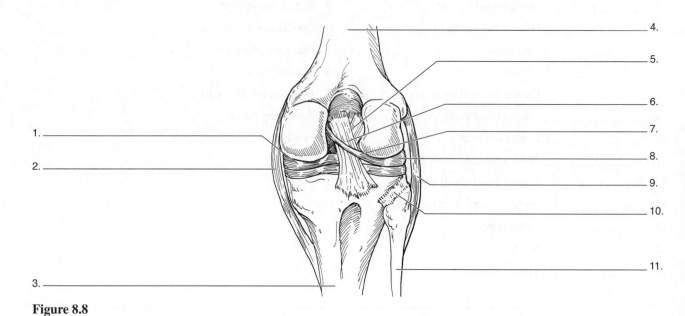

Figure 8.8

COMPLETE THE TABLE: LIGAMENTS

This activity will help you review the functions of the various ligaments.

INSTRUCTIONS. Fill in the missing information about ligaments of the pelvis, hip, and knee. The first column indicates a ligament of this region, the second identifies which bony landmarks it joins, and the third indicates the function of the ligament or what movements are limited by this structure. The first one is completed for you as an example.

Ligament	Bony Landmarks Joined	Function
Anterior cruciate	Medial tibial plateau Posterior surface of lateral femoral condyle	Limits anterior glide of tibia and posterior glide of femur
Anterior sacrococcygeal		
Anterior sacroiliac		
Iliofemoral		

(Continued on next page)

Ligament	Bony Landmarks Joined	Function
Iliolumbar		
Inguinal		
Ischiofemoral		
Lateral collateral		
Medial collateral		
Posterior cruciate		
Posterior meniscofemoral		
Posterior sacrococcygeal		
Posterior sacroiliac		
Proximal tibiofibular		
Pubofemoral		
Sacrospinous		
Sacrotuberous		

LABEL MUSCLES OF THE PELVIS, THIGH, AND KNEE

Besides maintaining posture, alignment, and balance, the large muscles in this region initiate walking, running, lifting, jumping, and other movements in the lower body. The following activities will help you become more familiar with these muscles.

INSTRUCTIONS. The following diagrams depict the superficial muscles of the pelvis, thigh, and knee. Label each of the following structures.

List of Structures, Anterior View

Adductor longus
Gracilis
Iliacus
Iliotibial band

Pectineus
Psoas
Rectus femoris
Sartorius

Tensor fascia latae
Vastus lateralis
Vastus medialis

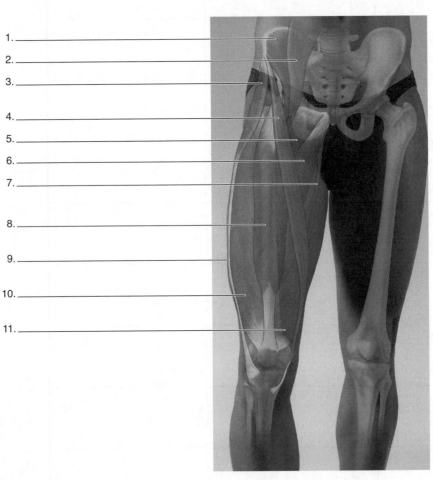

1. _____

2. _____

3. _____

4. _____

5. _____

6. _____

7. _____

8. _____

9. _____

10. _____

11. _____

Figure 8.9

List of Structures, Lateral View

Biceps femoris
(long head)
Biceps femoris
(short head)
Gluteus maximus
Gluteus medius
Iliotibial band
Rectus femoris
Sartorius
Tensor fascia latae
Vastus lateralis
(use twice)

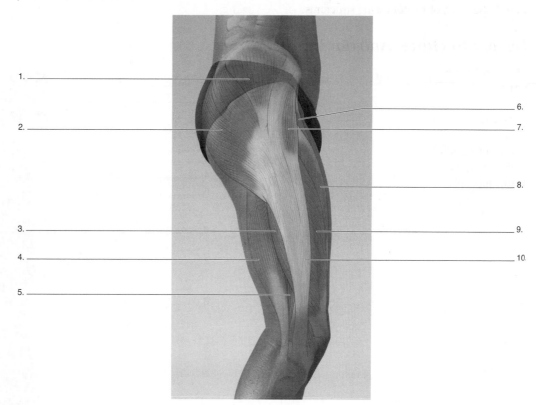

1. ___
2. ___
3. ___
4. ___
5. ___

6. ___
7. ___
8. ___
9. ___
10. ___

Figure 8.10

List of Structures, Posterior View

Adductor magnus
Biceps femoris (long head)
Biceps femoris (short head)
Gluteus maximus
Gluteus medius
Gracilis
Iliotibial band
Popliteus
Sartorius
Semimembranosus
Semitendinosus

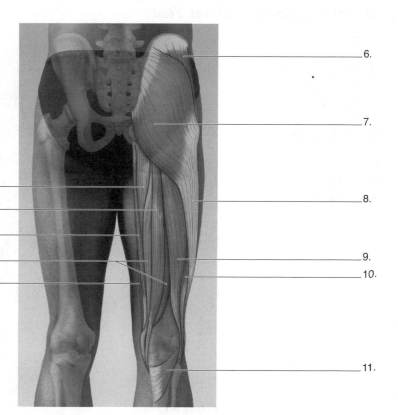

1. ___
2. ___
3. ___
4. ___
5. ___

6. ___
7. ___
8. ___
9. ___
10. ___
11. ___

Figure 8.11

INSTRUCTIONS. The following diagrams depict the deep muscles of the pelvis, thigh, and knee. Label each of the following structures.

List of Structures, Anterior View

Adductor longus
Gracilis
Iliacus
Pectineus
Psoas
Vastus intermedius
Vastus lateralis
Vastus medialis

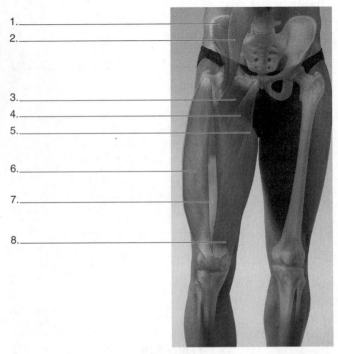

1._____
2._____

3._____
4._____
5._____

6._____

7._____

8._____

Figure 8.12

List of Structures, Lateral View

Biceps femoris
  (long head)
Biceps femoris
  (short head)
Gluteus medius
  (cut)
Gluteus minimus
Iliacus
Psoas
Rectus femoris
Vastus lateralis

1._____

2._____

3._____

4._____

5.
6.

7.

8.

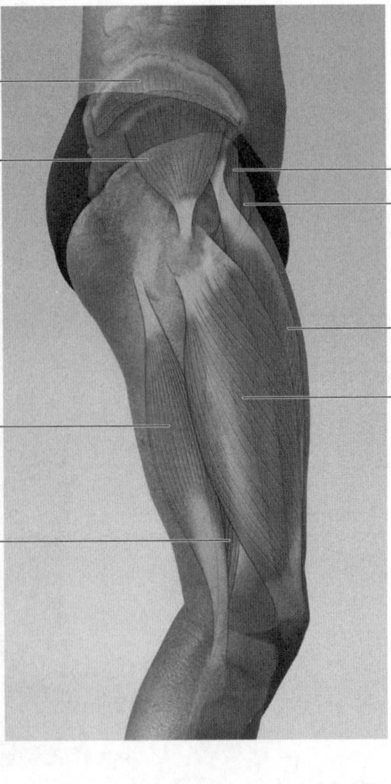

Figure 8.13

List of Structures, Posterior View

Biceps femoris (short head)   Gluteus medius (cut)   Piriformis
Gemellus inferior   Gluteus minimus   Quadratus femoris
Gemellus superior   Obturator internus   Semitendinosus

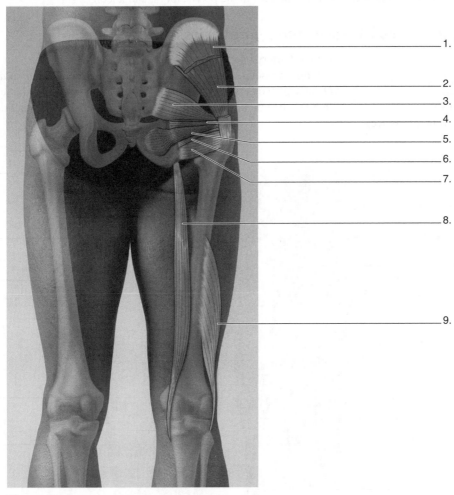

Figure 8.14

LABEL SPECIAL STRUCTURES

Several vulnerable structures are located both superficially and deep in the pelvis, thigh, and knee. Awareness of organs, blood vessels, lymph nodes and vessels, and nerves is critical when palpating and working in this area. Complete the following activities to help familiarize yourself with these structures.

INSTRUCTIONS. Label the following special structures in the pelvis, thigh, and knee.

List of Structures, Blood Vessels and Lymphatics, Anterior View

Anterior tibial artery
Deep inguinal nodes
Deep lymph vessels
Deep subinguinal node
Femoral artery and vein (use twice)

Femoral artery and vein and deep
  lymph vessels
Great saphenous vein (use twice)
Inguinal ligament

Popliteal nodes
Superficial inguinal nodes (use twice)
Superficial lymphatic vessels
Superficial subinguinal nodes

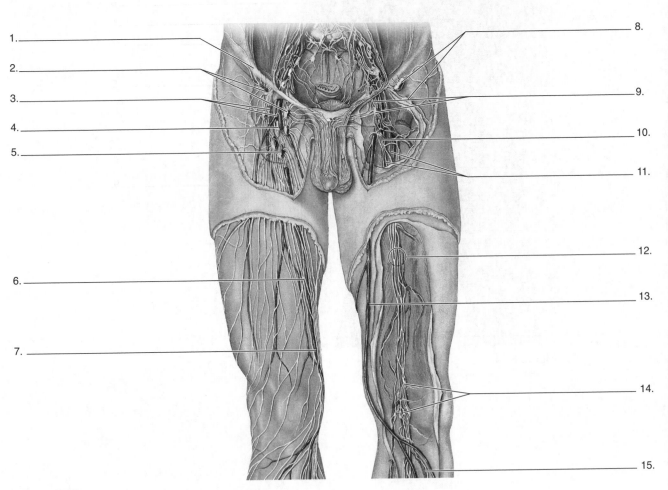

1.
2.
3.
4.
5.
6.
7.

8.
9.
10.
11.
12.
13.
14.
15.

Figure 8.15

List of Structures, Nerves Anterior View

Anterior cutaneous nerve
Common peroneal
  nerve
Deep peroneal nerve
Femoral nerve
Inguinal ligament

Lateral branch of anterior
  cutaneous nerve
Lateral femoral cutaneous nerve
Lumbar plexus
Medial branch of anterior cutaneous
  nerve

Obturator nerve
Rectus femoris muscle
Sacral plexus
Saphenous nerve
Superficial peroneal nerve

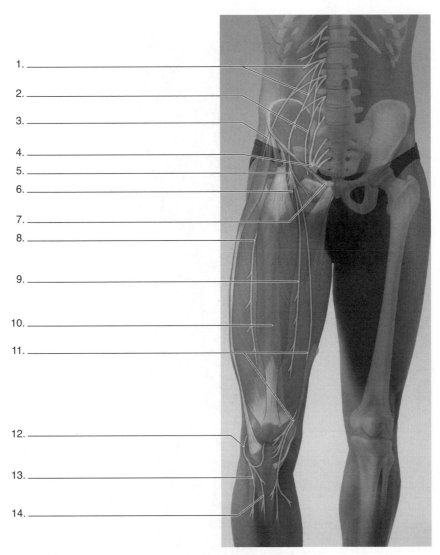

1. ———
2. ———
3. ———
4. ———
5. ———
6. ———
7. ———
8. ———
9. ———
10. ———
11. ———
12. ———
13. ———
14. ———

Figure 8.16

List of Structures, Nerves Posterior View

Biceps femoris muscle (long head cut)
Common peroneal nerve
First perforating artery
Fourth perforating artery
Gastrocnemius muscle
Gluteus minimus muscle
Inferior gluteal artery and nerve
Lateral sural cutaneous nerve

Medial circumflex femoral artery
Medial cluneal nerves
Medial sural cutaneous nerve
Muscular branches of sciatic nerve
Piriformis muscle
Popliteal artery and vein
Posterior cutaneous nerve
Sciatic nerve

Second and third perforating arteries
Semitendinosus muscle
Small saphenous vein
Superior cluneal nerves
Superior gluteal artery and nerve
Tibial nerve
Vastus lateralis muscle

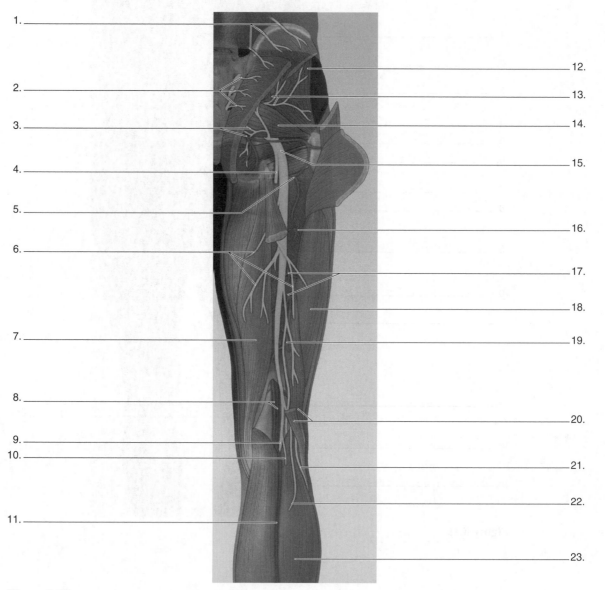

Figure 8.17

IDENTIFY HIP AND KNEE MOVEMENTS

The coxal joints and tibiofemoral joints work together to position the leg or the rest of the body over the leg.

INSTRUCTIONS. Beneath each of the following figures, write the name of each movement.

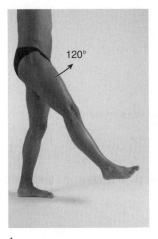 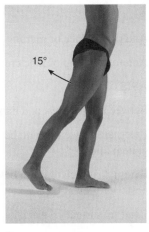 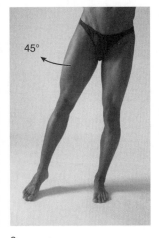 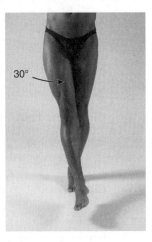

1._____   2._____   3._____   4._____

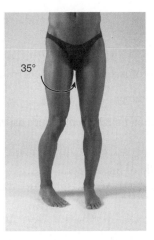 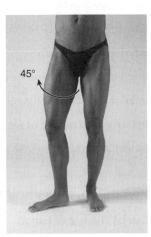

5._____   6._____   **Figure 8.18**

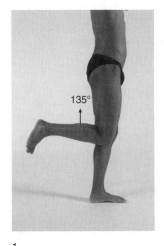 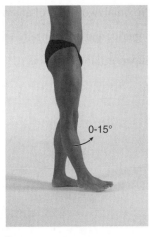 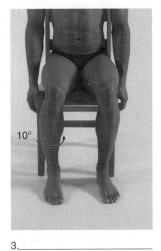 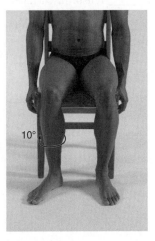

1._____   2._____   3._____   4._____

Figure 8.19

MATCH MUSCLE ORIGINS, INSERTIONS, AND ACTIONS

Each individual muscle in this region has unique muscle attachments, crosses a specific joint or joints, and performs specific movements.

INSTRUCTIONS. Match each muscle of the pelvis, thigh, and knee with the corresponding origin. Answers may be used more than one time.

1. _____ Adductor brevis
2. _____ Adductor longus
3. _____ Adductor magnus
4. _____ Biceps femoris
5. _____ Gluteus maximus
6. _____ Gluteus medius
7. _____ Gluteus minimus
8. _____ Gracilis
9. _____ Iliacus
10. _____ Inferior gemellus
11. _____ Obturator externus
12. _____ Obturator internus
13. _____ Pectineus
14. _____ Piriformis
15. _____ Popliteus
16. _____ Psoas
17. _____ Quadratus femoris
18. _____ Rectus femoris
19. _____ Sartorius
20. _____ Semimembranosus
21. _____ Semitendinosus
22. _____ Superior gemellus
23. _____ Tensor fascia latae
24. _____ Vastus intermedius
25. _____ Vastus lateralis
26. _____ Vastus medialis

A. AIIS

B. Anterior surface of sacrum

C. Anterolateral lip of iliac crest

D. ASIS

E. Between pubic crest and pubic symphysis

F. External surface of ilium between anterior and inferior gluteal lines

G. External surface of ilium between iliac crest and anterior and posterior gluteal lines

H. External surface of ischial spine

I. Greater trochanter, gluteal tuberosity, and proximal, lateral lip of linea aspera

J. Iliac fossa and ala of sacrum

K. Inferior ramus of pubis

L. Inferior ramus of pubis, ramus of ischium, ischial tuberosity

M. Interior surface of obturator foramen

N. Intertrochanteric line of femur and medial lip of linea aspera

O. Ischial tuberosity

P. Ischial tuberosity and lateral lip of linea aspera

Q. Lateral bodies and TVPs of T12–L5

R. Lateral condyle of femur

S. Outer surface of inferior ramus of pubis

T. Posterior iliac crest, posterior sacrum, coccyx, lumbar aponeurosis

U. Proximal two-thirds of anterior shaft of femur

V. Superior and inferior rami of pubis and ischium

W. Superior ramus of pubis

INSTRUCTIONS. Match each muscle of pelvis, thigh, and knee with the corresponding insertion.
Answers may be used more than once.

1. _____ Adductor brevis

2. _____ Adductor longus

3. _____ Adductor magnus

4. _____ Biceps femoris

5. _____ Gluteus maximus

6. _____ Gluteus medius

7. _____ Gluteus minimus

8. _____ Gracilis

9. _____ Iliacus

10. _____ Inferior gemellus

11. _____ Obturator externus

12. _____ Obturator internus

13. _____ Pectineus

14. _____ Piriformis

15. _____ Popliteus

16. _____ Psoas

17. _____ Quadratus femoris

18. _____ Rectus femoris

19. _____ Sartorius

20. _____ Semimembranosus

21. _____ Semitendinosus

22. _____ Superior gemellus

23. _____ Tensor fascia latae

24. _____ Vastus intermedius

25. _____ Vastus lateralis

26. _____ Vastus medialis

A. Anterior border of greater trochanter

B. Femoral crest, between greater and lesser trochanters

C. Fibular head and lateral condyle of tibia

D. Gluteal tuberosity of femur and lateral condyle of tibial via iliotibial band

E. Lateral condyle of tibia via iliotibial band

F. Lateral surface of greater trochanter

G. Lesser trochanter

H. Medial lip of linea aspera, medial supracondylar line, and adductor tubercle

I. Medial shaft of tibia via pes anserine tendon

J. Medial surface of greater trochanter

K. Middle one-third of medial lip of linea aspera

L. Pectineal line of femur

M. Pectineal line of femur and proximal one-half of medial lip of linea aspera

N. Posteromedial portion of medial condyle of tibia

O. Proximal posterior surface of tibia

P. Superior border of greater trochanter

Q. Tibial tuberosity via patellar tendon

R. Trochanteric fossa of femur

INSTRUCTIONS. Match each muscle of the pelvis, thigh, and knee with the corresponding actions. Choose all that apply. Some answers will be used more than once.

1. _____ Adductor brevis   A. Hip abduction

2. _____ Adductor longus   B. Hip adduction

3. _____ Adductor magnus   C. Hip extension

4. _____ Biceps femoris   D. Hip external rotation

5. _____ Gluteus maximus   E. Hip flexion

6. _____ Gluteus medius   F. Hip internal rotation

7. _____ Gluteus minimus   G. Knee extension

8. _____ Gracilis   H. Knee external rotation

9. _____ Iliacus   I. Knee flexion

10. _____ Inferior gemellus   J. Knee internal rotation

11. _____ Obturator externus

12. _____ Obturator internus

13. _____ Pectineus

14. _____ Piriformis

15. _____ Popliteus

16. _____ Psoas

17. _____ Quadratus femoris

18. _____ Rectus femoris

19. _____ Sartorius

20. _____ Semimembranosus

21. _____ Semitendinosus

22. _____ Superior gemellus

23. _____ Tensor fascia latae

24. _____ Vastus intermedius

25. _____ Vastus lateralis

26. _____ Vastus medialis

IDENTIFY SHORTENING AND LENGTHENING PELVIS, THIGH, AND KNEE MUSCLES

This activity will help you become more familiar with each muscle of the shoulder.

INSTRUCTIONS. For each of the following muscles, identify the position where the muscle is most shortened and the position that lengthens or stretches the muscle. The first one is completed as an example.

Adductor Brevis

Shortened position: adduct, flex, and externally rotate the hip

Lengthened position: abduct, extend, and internally rotate the hip

Adductor Longus and Pectineus

Shortened position: _____

_____

Lengthened position: _____

_____

Adductor Magnus

Shortened position: _____

_____

Lengthened position: _____

_____

Biceps Femoris, Semimembranosus, and Semitendinosus

Shortened position: _____

_____

Lengthened position: _____

_____

Gluteus Maximus

Shortened position: _____

_____

Lengthened position: _____

_____

Gluteus Medius and Minimus

Shortened position: _____

_____

Lengthened position: _____

_____

Gracilis

Shortened position: _____

_____

Lengthened position: _____

_____

Psoas and Iliacus

Shortened position: _____

_____

Lengthened position: _____

_____

Rectus Femoris

Shortened position: _____

_____

Lengthened position: _____

_____

Sartorius

Shortened position: _____

_____

Lengthened position: _____

_____

Tensor Fascia Latae

Shortened position: _____

_____

Lengthened position: _____

_____

Vastus Medialis, Intermedius, and Lateralis

Shortened position: _____

_____

Lengthened position: _____

_____

COMPLETE THE TABLE: SYNERGISTS/ANTAGONISTS

The following activity will help you gain a better sense of how the pelvic, thigh, and knee muscles work together or in opposition.

INSTRUCTIONS. Fill in the missing information about muscles of the pelvis, thigh, and knee. The first column indicates a movement of the hip or knee, the second identifies which muscles perform this action, and the third indicates the opposite action. The first one is completed for you as an example.

Movement	Muscles	Opposite Action
Hip abduction	Gluteus maximus (upper fibers) Gluteus medius Gluteus minimus Piriformis Sartorius Tensor fascia latae	
Hip adduction		
Hip extension		
Hip external rotation		
Hip flexion		

(*Continued on next page*)

Movement	Muscles	Opposite Action
Hip internal rotation		
Knee extension		
Knee external rotation		
Knee flexion		
Knee internal rotation		

PUTTING THE PELVIS, THIGH, AND KNEE IN MOTION

The following activity synthesizes all that you have learned about the pelvis, thigh, and knee. As in previous chapters, you will examine several specific movements: describe (1) the joints involved, (2) which joint motions occur, and (3) in what sequence these occur. It is often helpful to perform the movement yourself, observe someone else performing the movement, or watch an animation or video of the movement to better understand what is happening and when.

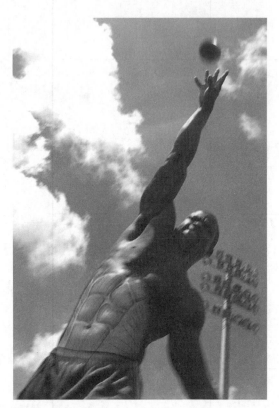

Figure 8.20 Shotput

INSTRUCTIONS. List the joints involved in the movement shown.

_____

_____

_____

INSTRUCTIONS. List the motions that occur at each joint.

_____

_____

_____

INSTRUCTIONS. List the sequence of events involved in the movement shown.

_____

_____

_____

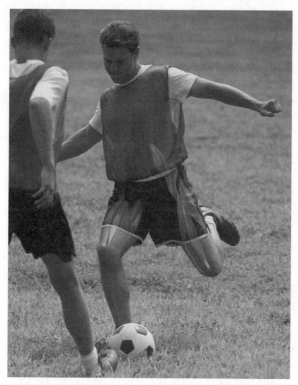

Figure 8.21 Kicking

INSTRUCTIONS. List the joints involved in the movement shown.

_____

_____

_____

INSTRUCTIONS. List the motions that occur at each joint.

_____

_____

_____

INSTRUCTIONS. List the sequence of events involved in the movement shown.

_____

_____

_____

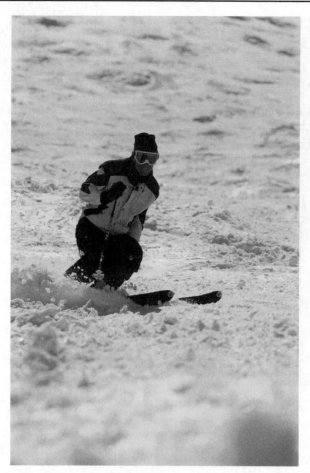

Figure 8.22 Downhill Skiing

INSTRUCTIONS. List the joints involved in the movement shown.

_____

_____

_____

INSTRUCTIONS. List the motions that occur at each joint.

_____

_____

_____

INSTRUCTIONS. List the sequence of events involved in the movement shown.

_____

_____

_____

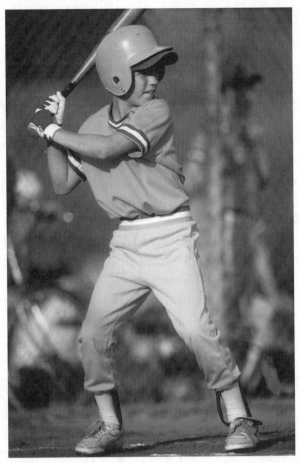

Figure 8.23 Baseball Swing

INSTRUCTIONS. List the joints involved in the movement shown.

_____

_____

_____

INSTRUCTIONS. List the motions that occur at each joint.

_____

_____

_____

INSTRUCTIONS. List the sequence of events involved in the movement shown.

_____

_____

_____

WORD CHALLENGE

This final exercise checks your recall of terms and concepts introduced throughout the chapter.

INSTRUCTIONS. Complete the crossword using the following clues.

ACROSS:

1. Basin-shaped cavity formed by the sacrum, coccyx, and coxal bone.
5. Has a crest, a fossa, and anterior and posterior spines.
6. Hyperextension of the knee can damage this muscle.
8. Modified hinge joint that includes articulations between the femur, tibia, and patella. Knee cap.
9. Latin for "huge."
10. Large nerve running inferiorly along the thigh.
12. Thigh bone.
14. Name reflects the Latin word for "twin."
15. Postural deviation in which the knee "opens" laterally.

DOWN:

1. Its "goose foot" shape is formed by the insertion of the sartorius, gracilis, and semitendinosus muscles.
2. Latin for "smallest."
3. Lateral hamstring muscle.
4. Extends, externally rotates, abducts, and adducts the hip.
6. Origin of this muscle is T12–L5 and insertion is lesser trochanter of femur.
7. Longest muscle in the human body.
11. Bony landmark anterior and inferior to the iliac crest.
12. Lateral bone of the leg.
13. Knee cap.

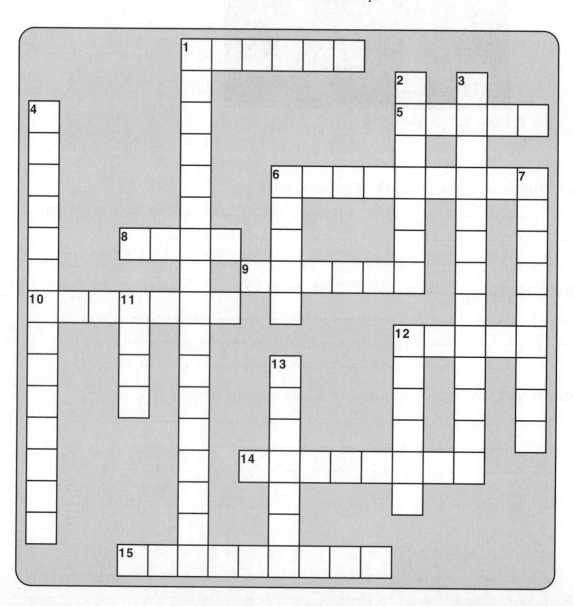

Leg, Ankle, and Foot

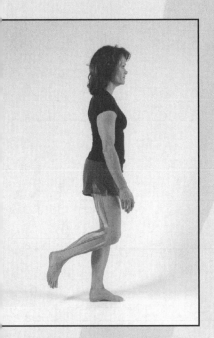

Our final segment moves distally to the leg, ankle, and foot. The complex architecture of the foot provides an adaptable surface that also distributes force and absorbs shock when functioning properly. The ankle directs tremendous power into the leg, initiating explosive movements such as running and jumping. The following activities will help you better understand the structure and function of the leg, ankle, and foot.

LABEL SURFACE LANDMARKS

This activity will assist you in orienting yourself during palpation and visually assessing the health and function of underlying structures.

INSTRUCTIONS. The following images depict the major surface landmarks of the leg and foot. Label each of the following in the spaces provided.

List of Structures, Anterior View

Extensor digitorum longus
   muscle
Fibular head
Gastrocnemius muscle

Lateral malleolus
Medial malleolus
Peroneus longus muscle
Shaft of tibia

Soleus muscle
Tendon of tibialis
   anterior
Tibialis anterior muscle

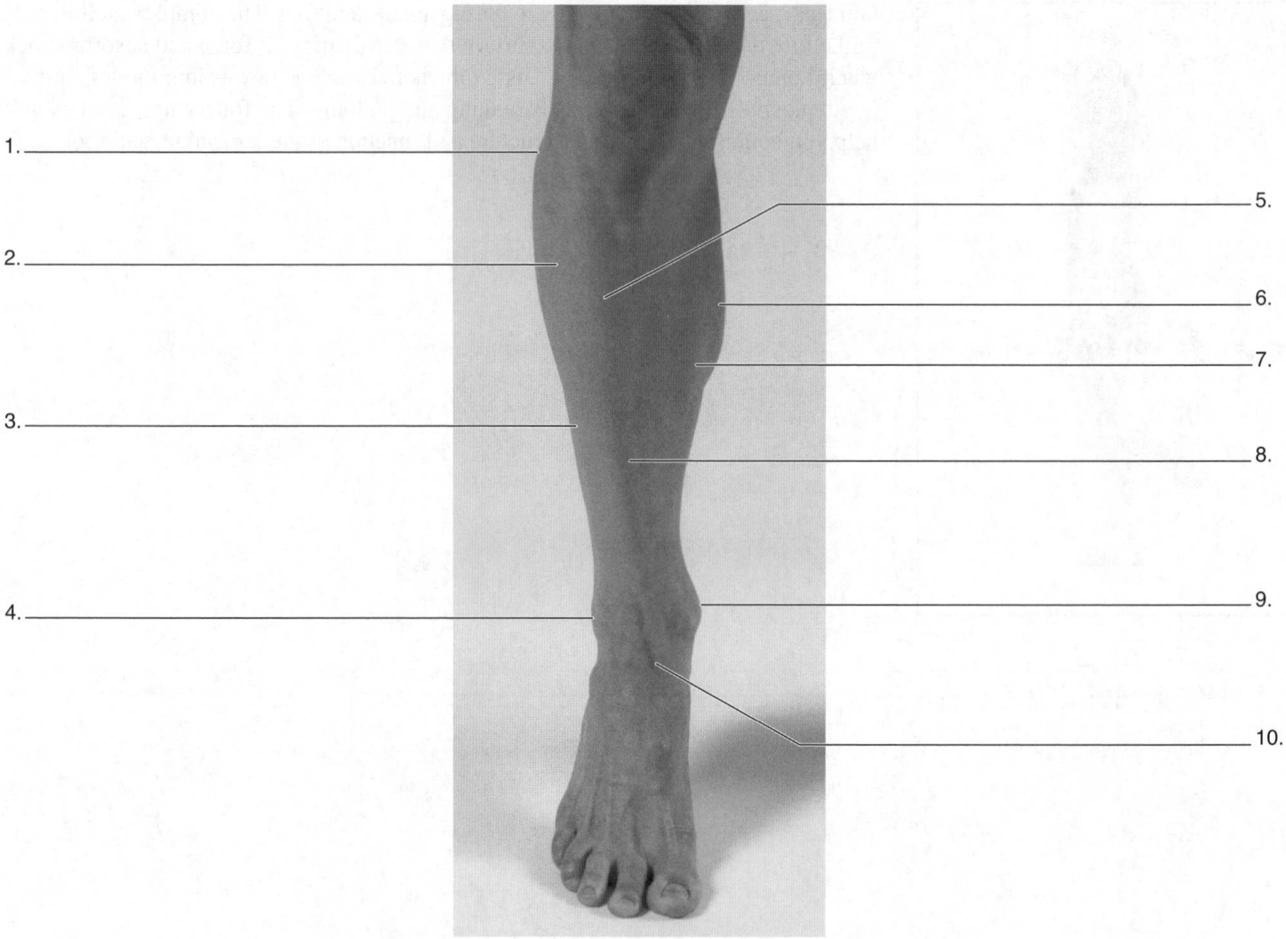

1. _____

2. _____

3. _____

4. _____

5. _____

6. _____

7. _____

8. _____

9. _____

10. _____

Figure 9.1

List of Structures, Lateral View

Achilles tendon
Extensor digitorum longus muscle
Extensor digitorum longus tendons

Gastrocnemius muscle
Head of fibula
Peroneus longus muscle

Peroneus longus tendon
Soleus muscle
Tibialis anterior muscle

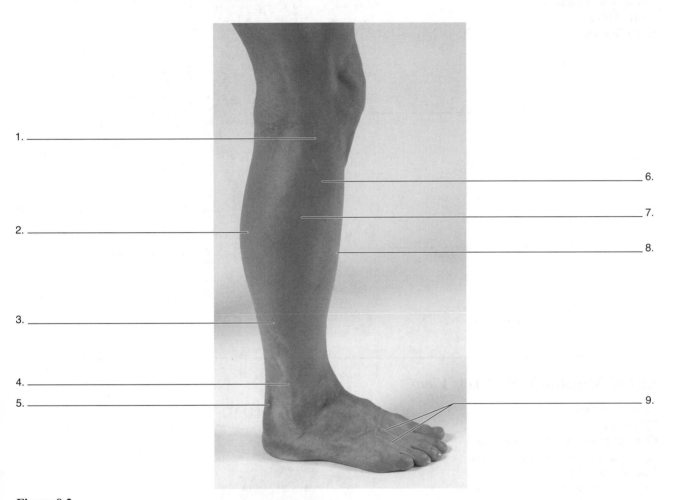

1. _____

2. _____

3. _____

4. _____

5. _____

6. _____

7. _____

8. _____

9. _____

Figure 9.2

List of Structures, Medial View

Achilles tendon
Calcaneus
Extensor hallucis longus tendon
Gastrocnemius muscle (medial head)
Medial longitudinal arch
Shaft of tibia
Soleus muscle

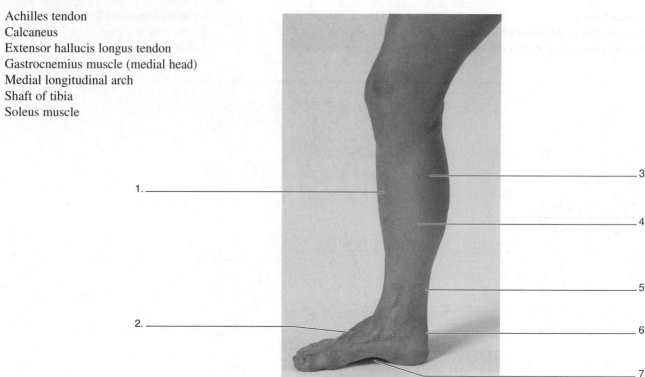

1. ____
2. ____

3. ____
4. ____
5. ____
6. ____
7. ____

Figure 9.3

List of Structures, Posterior View

Achilles tendon
Calcaneus
Gastrocnemius muscle (lateral head)
Gastrocnemius muscle (medial head)
Lateral edge of soleus
Lateral malleolus
Medial edge of
   soleus muscle
Medial malleolus

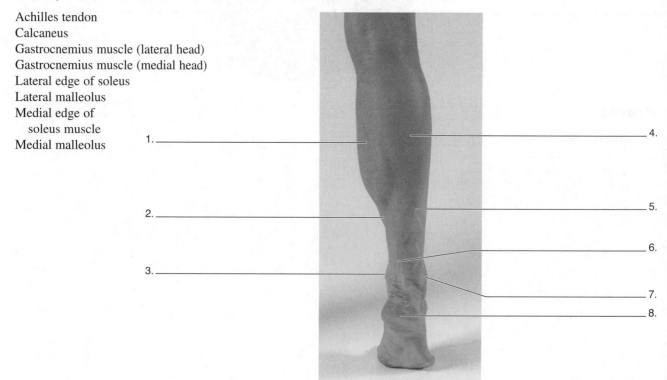

1. ____
2. ____
3. ____

4. ____
5. ____
6. ____
7. ____
8. ____

Figure 9.4

COLOR AND LABEL SKELETAL STRUCTURES

Bones and bony landmarks provide consistent touchstones as we locate, differentiate, and explore soft-tissue structures such as muscles, tendons, and ligaments in the leg, ankle, and foot.

INSTRUCTIONS. The following images depict the bones and bony landmarks for the leg, ankle, and foot. Color and label each of the following structures.

List of Structures, Anterior View

Calcaneus
Cuboid
Distal phalanx
Distal tibiofibular
  joint
Fibular head
Fibular shaft

Fifth metatarsal
First metatarsal
Lateral condyle of tibia
Lateral malleolus
Medial condyle of tibia
Medial malleolus
Middle phalanx

Proximal phalanx
Proximal tibiofibular
  joint
Talocrural joint
Tarsals
Tibial shaft
Tibial tuberosity

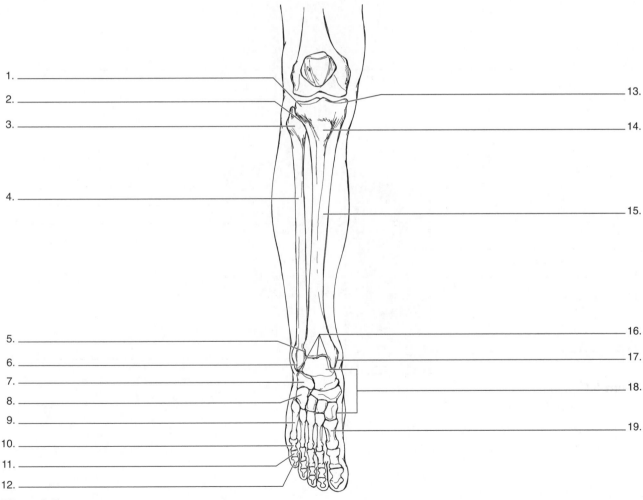

1. _____
2. _____
3. _____
4. _____
5. _____
6. _____
7. _____
8. _____
9. _____
10. _____
11. _____
12. _____

13. _____
14. _____
15. _____
16. _____
17. _____
18. _____
19. _____

Figure 9.5

List of Structures, Posterior View

Calcaneus
Cuboid
Cuneiforms
Distal phalanx
Fibula
Lateral malleolus

Medial malleolus
Metatarsals
Middle phalanx
Navicular
Neck of fibula

Proximal phalanx
Soleal line
Subtalar joint
Talus (use twice)
Tibia

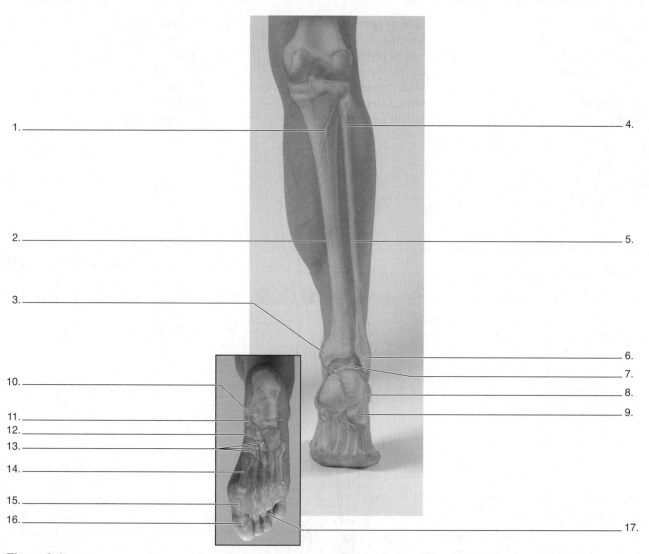

1. _____

2. _____

3. _____

10. _____

11. _____
12. _____
13. _____

14. _____

15. _____
16. _____

4. _____

5. _____

6. _____
7. _____
8. _____
9. _____

17. _____

Figure 9.6

List of Structures, Foot, Lateral View

Attachment of calcaneofibular
  ligament
Calcaneus
Cuboid

Cuneiforms
Lateral tubercle talus
Metatarsals
Navicular

Peroneal tubercle
Phalanges
Talus: body, head, neck (label each)
Tuberosity of fifth metatarsal

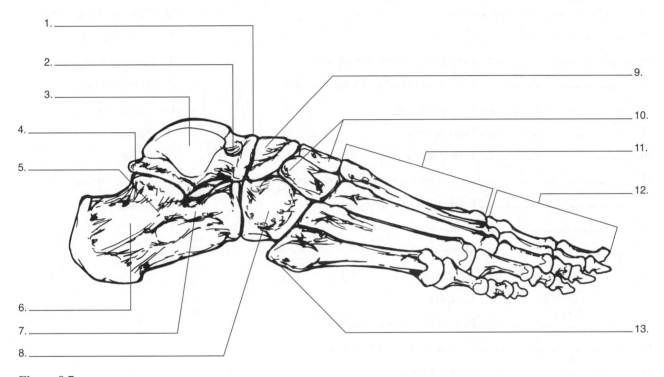

Figure 9.7

INSTRUCTIONS. Match each of the following bony landmarks with the corresponding muscle attachment. Choose all that apply. Answers may be used more than once.

1. _____ Anterior fibula

2. _____ Base of fifth metatarsal

3. _____ Calcaneus via Achilles tendon

4. _____ Cuboid

5. _____ Cuneiforms

6. _____ First distal phalanx, dorsal surface

7. _____ First distal phalanx, plantar surface

8. _____ First metatarsal

9. _____ Head of fibula

10. _____ Lateral fibula

11. _____ Lateral supracondylar line of femur

12. _____ Lateral tibial condyle

13. _____ Medial cuneiform

14. _____ Medial fibula

15. _____ Metatarsals 2–4

16. _____ Navicular

17. _____ Phalanges 2–5, dorsal surface

18. _____ Phalanges 2–5, plantar surface

19. _____ Posterior fibula

20. _____ Posterior surface of lateral femoral condyle

21. _____ Posterior surface of medial femoral condyle

22. _____ Posterior tibia

23. _____ Soleal line and posterior surface of tibia

A. Extensor digitorum longus

B. Extensor hallucis longus

C. Flexor digitorum longus

D. Flexor hallucis longus

E. Gastrocnemius

F. Peroneus brevis

G. Peroneus longus

H. Peroneus tertius

I. Plantaris

J. Soleus

K. Tibialis anterior

L. Tibialis posterior

LABEL JOINTS AND LIGAMENTS

The leg offers tremendous stability while the joints of the ankle and foot move in various combinations. This next activity will help you explore the joints of the leg, ankle, and foot and the ligaments that hold them together.

INSTRUCTIONS. The following images depict the bones and ligaments of the leg, ankle, and foot. Label the following structures.

List of Structures, Foot, Lateral View

Anterior talofibular ligament	Calcaneofibular ligament	Long plantar ligament
Anterior tibiotalar ligament	Cuneometatarsal ligaments	Posterior talofibular ligament
Bifurcate ligament	Dorsal cuneiform ligaments	Talonavicular ligament
Calcaneocuboid ligament	Dorsal metatarsal ligaments	Tarsometatarsal ligaments

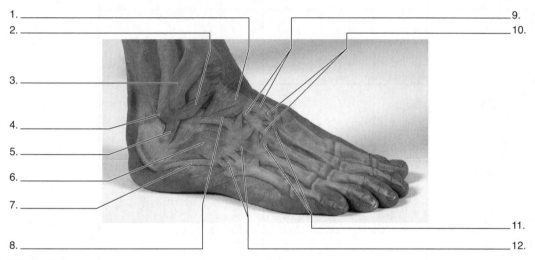

Figure 9.8

List of Structures, Foot, Medial View

Anterior tibiotalar ligament	Dorsal tarsometatarsal ligaments	Posterior tibiotalar ligament
Calcaneus	Medial talocalcaneal ligament	Tibia
Dorsal cuneonavicular ligaments	Plantar calcaneonavicular ligament	Tibiocalcaneal ligament
Dorsal talonavicular ligament	Posterior talocalcaneal ligament	Tibionavicular ligament

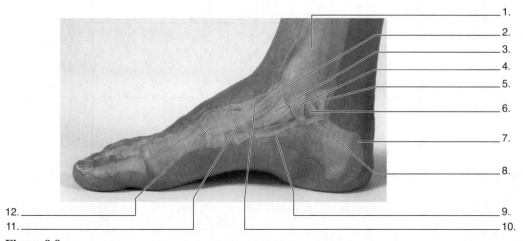

Figure 9.9

COMPLETE THE TABLE: LIGAMENTS

This activity will help you review the functions of the various ligaments.

INSTRUCTIONS. Fill in the missing information about ligaments of the leg, ankle, and foot. The first column indicates a ligament of this region, the second identifies which bony landmarks it joins, and the third indicates the function of the ligament or what movements are limited by this structure. The first one is completed for you as an example.

Ligament	Bony Landmarks Joined	Function
Anterior talofibular	Distal fibula Lateral neck of talus	Limits forward glide of talus
Bifurcate		
Calcaneofibular		
Deltoid		
Long plantar		
Medial talocalcaneal		
Posterior inferior talofibular		
Plantar calcaneonavicular ligament		
Tibiofibular		

LABEL MUSCLES OF THE LEG, ANKLE, AND FOOT

Strong muscles pull the ball of the foot against the ground, driving the body forward and up. Muscles on the front and sides of the ankle and foot work together to maintain joint alignment, balance the body over the foot, direct movement, or control force distribution across the foot. The following activities will help you become more familiar with these muscles.

INSTRUCTIONS. The following diagrams depict the superficial muscles of the leg, ankle, and foot. Label each of the following structures.

List of Structures, Anterior View

Extensor digitorum longus	Peroneus brevis	Soleus
Extensor hallucis longus	Peroneus longus	Tibialis anterior
Gastrocnemius		

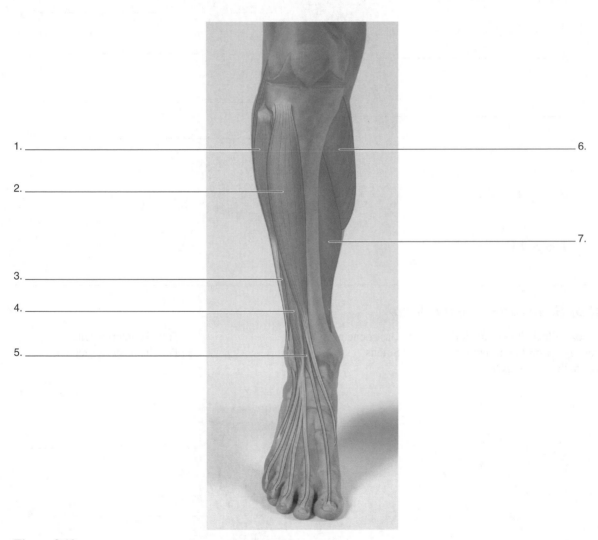

1. _____   6. ___

2. _____

7. ___

3. _____

4. _____

5. _____

Figure 9.10

List of Structures, Lateral View

Abductor digiti minimi
Extensor digitorum longus
Extensor hallucis longus
Gastrocnemius

Peroneus brevis
Peroneus longus
Peroneus tertius
Plantaris

Soleus
Tibialis anterior

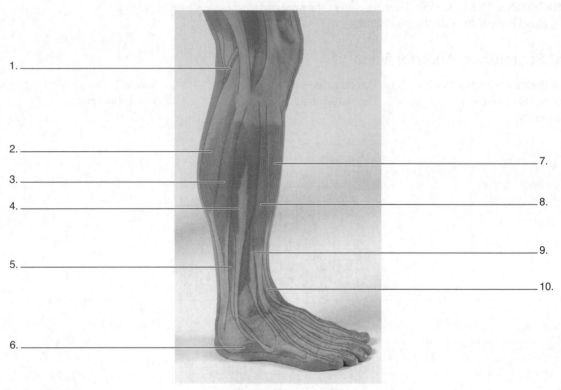

Figure 9.11

List of Structures, Medial View

Extensor hallucis longus tendon
Flexor digitorum longus tendon
Flexor hallucis longus tendon

Gastrocnemius
Soleus

Tibialis anterior tendon
Tibialis posterior tendon

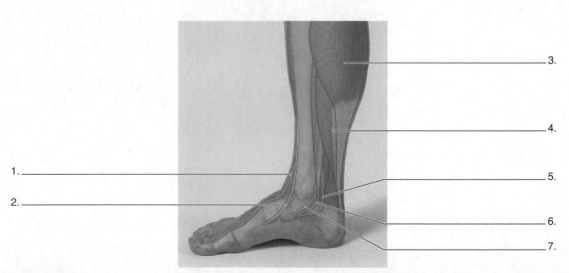

Figure 9.12

INSTRUCTIONS. The following diagrams depict the deep muscles of the leg, ankle, and foot. Label each of the following structures.

List of Structures, Posterior View

Flexor digitorum longus
Flexor hallucis longus
Peroneus brevis
Peroneus longus
Popliteus muscle
Tibialis posterior

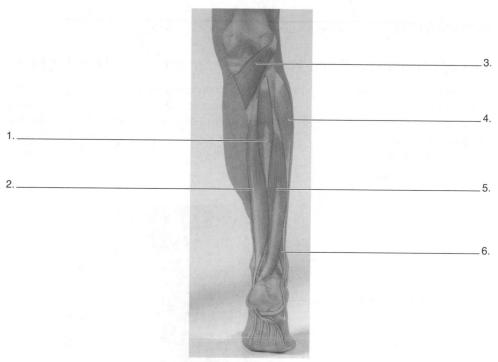

Figure 9.13

List of Structures, Foot, Plantar View

Abductor digiti
  minimi muscle
Abductor hallucis
  muscle
Calcaneus
Flexor digiti minimi
  brevis muscle
Flexor digitorum
  brevis muscle
Flexor digitorum
  longus tendons
Flexor hallucis
  longus tendon
Flexor hallucis
  brevis muscle
Lumbrical muscles
Plantar aponeurosis
  (cut)
Plantar interosseous
  muscle

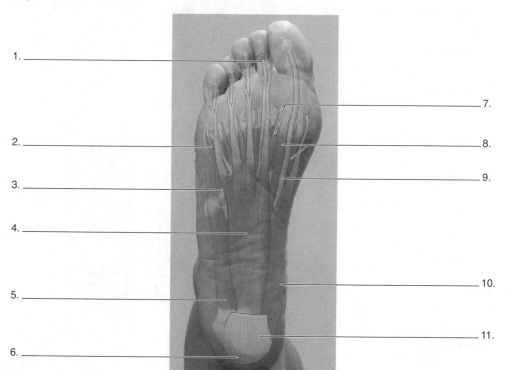

Figure 9.14

LABEL SPECIAL STRUCTURES

Several vulnerable structures are located in the back of the knee and medial leg. To safely and effectively work in this area, you must have a clear understanding of where these are located. The following activities will help familiarize you with these structures and their locations.

INSTRUCTIONS. Label the following special structures of the leg and foot.

List of Structures, Blood Vessels and Lymphatics, Anterior View

Anterior tibial artery, vein,
and lymph vessels
Anterior tibial node
Deep lymph vessels
Dorsal venous arch

Dorsalis pedis artery, vein,
and lymph vessels
Great saphenous vein (use twice)
Peroneal artery, veins, and lymph nodes
Popliteal nodes

Posterior tibial artery, vein,
and lymph vessels
Posterior tibial node
Small saphenous vein
and lymph nodes

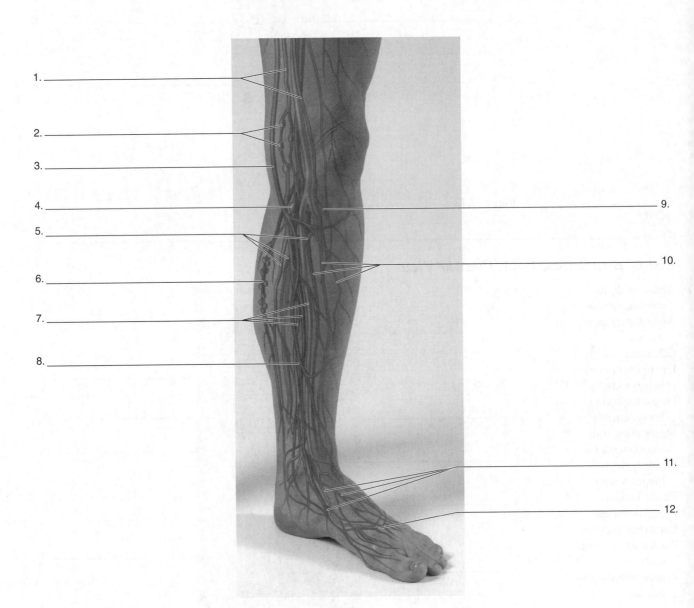

1. _____
2. _____
3. _____
4. _____
5. _____
6. _____
7. _____
8. _____

9. _____
10. _____
11. _____
12. _____

Figure 9.15

List of Structures, Blood Vessels and Lymphatics, Posterior View

Common fibular
 (peroneal) nerve
Popliteal artery
 and vein
Popliteal lymph nodes
Small saphenous vein

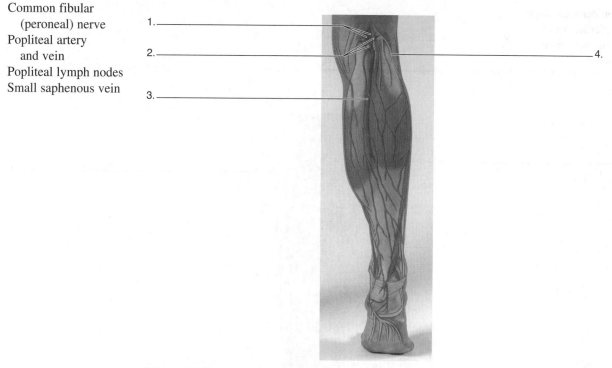

Figure 9.16

List of Structures, Nerves, Anterior View

Anterior tibial artery
Deep peroneal nerve
Intermedial dorsal
 branch of superficial
 peroneal nerve
Lateral branch of deep
 peroneal nerve
Medial dorsal
 cutaneous
 branch of
 superficial
 peroneal nerve
Saphenous nerve
Superficial peroneal
 nerve
Sural nerve

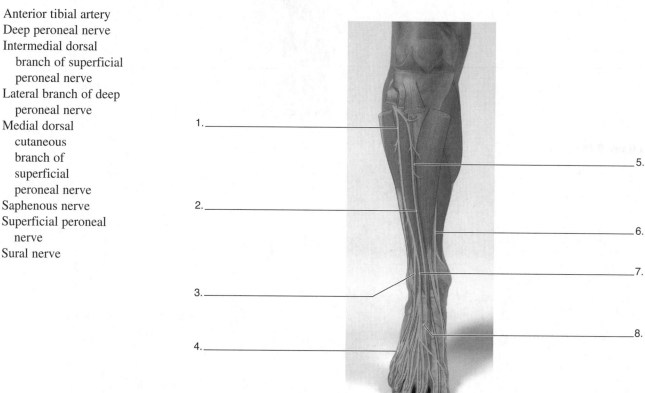

Figure 9.17

List of Structures, Nerves, Posterior View

Common peroneal nerve
Lateral plantar nerve
Medial plantar nerve
Tibial nerve

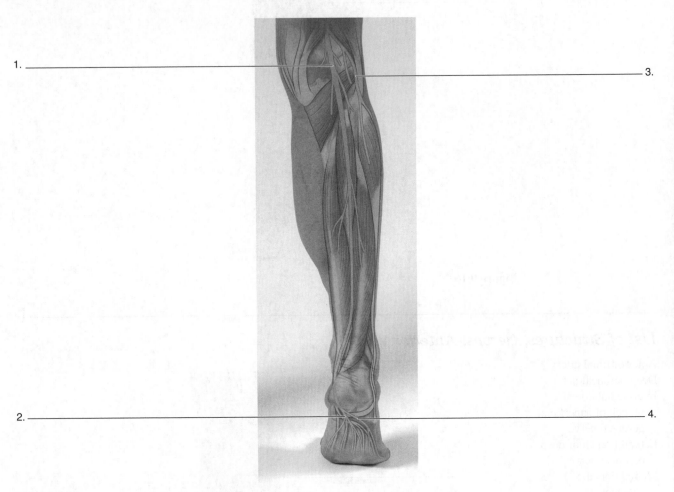

1. _____

2. _____

3. _____

4. _____

Figure 9.18

IDENTIFY ANKLE AND FOOT MOVEMENTS

The talocrural joint, subtalar joint, and small additional joints of the leg and foot work together to initiate or drive motion from the foot, position the foot, or stabilize the rest of the body over the foot.

INSTRUCTIONS. Beneath each of the following figures, write the name of each movement.

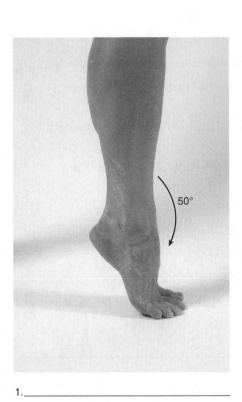

1._____

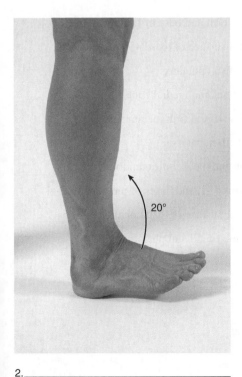

2._____

Figure 9.19

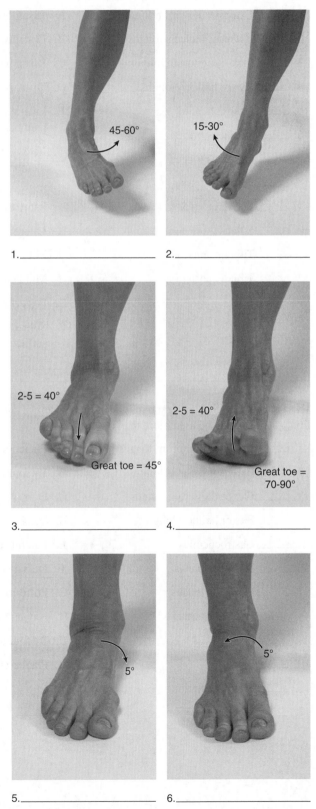

1._____   2._____

3._____   4._____

5._____   6._____

Figure 9.20

MATCH MUSCLE ORIGINS, INSERTIONS, AND ACTIONS

Each muscle has unique muscle attachments, crosses a specific joint or joints, and performs specific movements.

INSTRUCTIONS. Match each muscle of the leg, ankle, and foot with the corresponding origin. Use each answer one time.

1. _____ Extensor digitorum longus

2. _____ Extensor hallucis longus

3. _____ Flexor digitorum longus

4. _____ Flexor hallucis longus

5. _____ Gastrocnemius

6. _____ Peroneus brevis

7. _____ Peroneus longus

8. _____ Peroneus tertius

9. _____ Plantaris

10. _____ Soleus

11. _____ Tibialis anterior

12. _____ Tibialis posterior

A. Distal one-third of anterior surface of fibula and interosseous membrane

B. Distal two-thirds of lateral surface of fibula

C. Distal part of lateral supracondylar line of femur

D. Distal posterior surface of fibula and interosseous membrane

E. Lateral condyle and proximal one-half of tibia and interosseous membrane

F. Lateral condyle of tibia, proximal anterior fibula, and interosseous membrane

G. Lateral posterior tibia, proximal two-thirds of medial fibula and interosseous membrane

H. Lateral two-thirds and head of the fibula

I. Middle of anterior surface of fibula and interosseous membrane

J. Middle of posterior surface of tibia

K. Posterior surface of medial and lateral femoral condyles

L. Soleal line and posterior surface of tibia and posterior head and proximal surface of fibula

---

INSTRUCTIONS. Match each muscle of the leg, ankle, and foot with the corresponding insertion. Answers may be used more than once.

1. _____ Extensor digitorum longus

2. _____ Extensor hallucis longus

3. _____ Flexor digitorum longus

4. _____ Flexor hallucis longus

5. _____ Gastrocnemius

6. _____ Peroneus brevis

7. _____ Peroneus longus

8. _____ Peroneus tertius

9. _____ Plantaris

10. _____ Soleus

11. _____ Tibialis anterior

12. _____ Tibialis posterior

A. Plantar surface of medial cuneiform and base of first metatarsal

B. By four tendons onto the dorsal surface of toes 2–5

C. Dorsal surface of base of first distal phalanx

D. Lateral sides of the first metatarsal and medial cuneiform

E. Lateral side of tuberosity at base of the fifth metatarsal

F. Dorsal surface of base of the fifth metatarsal

G. Posterior surface of calcaneous via the Achilles tendon

H. Navicular tuberosity, cuneiforms 1–3, and bases of metatarsals 2–4

I. By four tendons onto the plantar surface of distal phalanges 2–5

J. Plantar surface of the base of the first distal phalanx

INSTRUCTIONS. Match each muscle of the leg, ankle, and foot with the corresponding actions. Choose all that apply. Some answers will be used more than once.

1. _____ Extensor digitorum longus

2. _____ Extensor hallucis longus

3. _____ Flexor digitorum longus

4. _____ Flexor hallucis longus

5. _____ Gastrocnemius

6. _____ Peroneus brevis

7. _____ Peroneus longus

8. _____ Peroneus tertius

9. _____ Plantaris

10. _____ Soleus

11. _____ Tibialis anterior

12. _____ Tibialis posterior

A. Plantarflexion

B. Dorsiflexion

C. Inversion

D. Eversion

E. Toe flexion

F. Toe extension

IDENTIFY SHORTENING AND LENGTHENING LEG, ANKLE, AND FOOT MUSCLES

This activity will help you become more familiar with the muscles of the leg, ankle, and foot.

INSTRUCTIONS. For each of the following muscles, identify the position where the muscle is most shortened and the position that lengthens or stretches the muscle. The first one is completed as an example.

Extensor Digitorum Longus

Shortened position: extend toes 2–4 at metacarpal and intercarpal joints, dorsiflex the ankle, and evert the foot

Lengthened position: flex toes 2–4 at metacarpal and inter-carpal joints, plantarflex the ankle, and invert the foot

Extensor Hallucis Longus

Shortened position: _____

_____

Lengthened position: _____

_____

Flexor Digitorum Longus

Shortened position: _____

_____

Lengthened position: _____

_____

Flexor Hallucis Longus

Shortened position: _____

_____

Lengthened position: _____

_____

Gastrocnemius

Shortened position: _____

_____

Lengthened position: _____

_____

Peroneus Brevis

Shortened position: _____

_____

Lengthened position: _____

_____

Peroneus Longus

Shortened position: _____

_____

Lengthened position: _____

_____

Peroneus Tertius

Shortened position: _____

_____

Lengthened position: _____

_____

Plantaris

Shortened position: _____

_____

Lengthened position: _____

_____

Soleus

Shortened position: _____

_____

Lengthened position: _____

_____

Tibialis Anterior

Shortened position: _____

_____

Lengthened position: _____

_____

Tibialis Posterior

Shortened position: _____

_____

Lengthened position: _____

_____

COMPLETE THE TABLE: SYNERGISTS/ANTAGONISTS

The following activity will help you consider how the muscles of the leg, ankle, and foot work together or in opposition.

INSTRUCTIONS. Fill in the missing information about muscles of the leg, ankle, and foot. The first column indicates a movement of the ankle or foot, the second identifies which muscles perform this action, and the third indicates the opposite action. The first one is completed for you as an example.

Movement	Muscles	Opposite Action
Dorsiflexion	Extensor digitorum longus Extensor hallucis longus Peroneus tertius Tibialis anterior	Plantarflexion
Eversion		
Inversion		
Plantarflexion		
Toe extension		
Toe flexion		

PUTTING THE LEG, ANKLE, AND FOOT IN MOTION

The following activity brings together all that you have learned about the leg, ankle, and foot. As you examine the following movements, describe: (1) which joints are involved, (2) which joint motions occur, and (3) in what sequence these occur.

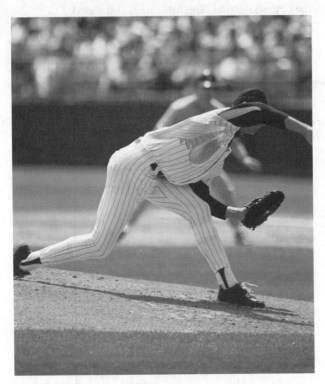

Figure 9.21 Overhand Throw

INSTRUCTIONS. List the joints involved in the movement shown.

_____

_____

_____

INSTRUCTIONS. List the motions that occur at each joint.

_____

_____

_____

INSTRUCTIONS. List the sequence of events involved in the movement shown.

_____

_____

_____

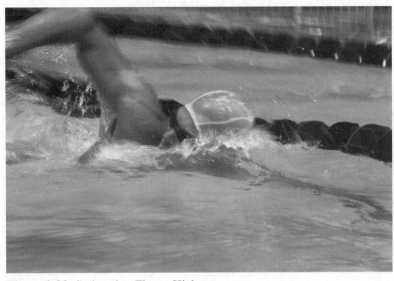

Figure 9.22 Swimming Flutter Kick

INSTRUCTIONS. List the joints involved in the movement shown.

_____

_____

_____

INSTRUCTIONS. List the motions that occur at each joint.

_____

_____

_____

INSTRUCTIONS. List the sequence of events involved in the movement shown.

_____

_____

_____

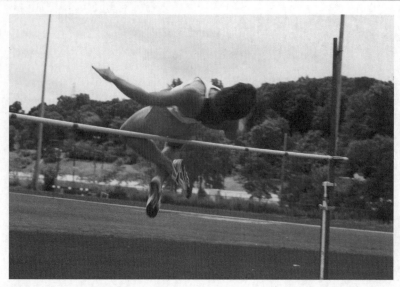

Figure 9.23 High Jump

INSTRUCTIONS. List the joints involved in the movement shown.

_____

_____

_____

INSTRUCTIONS. List the motions that occur at each joint.

_____

_____

_____

INSTRUCTIONS. List the sequence of events involved in the movement shown.

_____

_____

_____

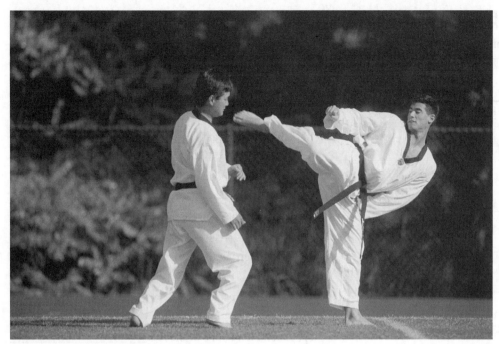

Figure 9.24 Karate Thrust Kick

INSTRUCTIONS. List the joints involved in the movement shown.

_____

_____

_____

INSTRUCTIONS. List the motions that occur at each joint.

_____

_____

_____

INSTRUCTIONS. List the sequence of events involved in the movement shown.

_____

_____

_____

WORD CHALLENGE

This final exercise checks your recall of terms and concepts introduced throughout the chapter.

INSTRUCTIONS. Twenty terms introduced in this chapter are hidden in the word search puzzle. Locate each term and write it next to its numbered definition. Terms may be found horizontally, vertically, or diagonally.

List of Terms

1. Flatfoot. _____

2. The main function of this muscle is to extend the great toe. _____

3. The name of this muscle is from the Latin word for bottom. _____

4. Happens when you stand on the ball of your foot.

   _____

5. Complex movement requiring participation of the upper and lower extremities, spine, and pelvis._____

   _____

6. Small muscles that flex the proximal phalanges. _____

   _____

7. Most superior tarsal bone. _____

   _____

8. Toe bone. _____

9. Two-headed calf muscle. _____

   _____

10. Tarsal bone of the heel. _____

    _____

11. Medial prominence on the distal tibia. _____

    _____

12. Hinge joint of ankle. _____

13. Medial long bone of the leg. _____

    _____

14. Long pennate muscle of the lateral leg. _____

    _____

15. Term referring to the top of the foot. _____

    _____

16. Latin for great toe. _____

    _____

17. Lateral long bone of the leg. _____

    _____

18. Band of connective tissue supporting the arch of the foot.

    _____

19. Continuation of the femoral artery of the thigh. _____

    _____

20. "Bump" below the knee. _____

    _____

```
O S P Q T U N J R I S P T M E B Z M N M S N
A P R R X F O Q V D Y T I B U G H T E V T H
G F G X M P J G P D T W B I D A O W M U R W
P D E V B R Y P F L M H I U Z O I X H Y Z J
D U L X M W O L F L T O A Z A X J Z T X S G
J F H Q I P P I P C A B L B U W T N P B U Q
A E H B G D P V A I B I T Q Q B H C C S G S
P L A N T A R A P O N E U R O S I S N G N B
G Y L R X M E I U Z R V B Z O S M K J J O S
A W L G N K O G D X D S E M O G F P B T L O
Y P U X A G P B J P U E R H P P T E X Y S Q
V V X R L I A J R N D G O R G K Z R J B I Q
U U D B A C T Q A T L S S H Y W U O G T C B
Y R M V H R H L U M B R I C A L S N P B U R
F Q G Z P R P K O Y V H T B X C P E W O L T
F T H R O S U E L O S E Y G K C F U L F L O
B J P M E D I A L M A L L E O L U S Q Q A B
D E U P L A N T A R F L E X I O N L B Z H L
P O P L I T E A L A R T E R Y C X O R B R W
X Q R C T W V L F I I A M E P R S N Z A O O
X X G S Y Z E O J Y G L Z J P Y T G Z D S F
F J D Q A X P C E V L U T I A X Y U K F N K
X Z N U P L I R N Q J S W S A L I S K P E P
A A F P W S E U E R Y S H Z A P U G Y I T K
B X N G A S T R O C N E M I U S S B U L X U
U T Z E B A C A L C A N E U S O W A I S E A
R C Y M S O X L W X Q Z Y I V T X Y D F S M
W S Z M H O B I D C H I C K C E Q F R E Q O
```

Answer Key

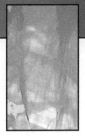

CHAPTER 1

Identify Regions and Directions

Figure 1.1, p. 2
1. Cranial
2. Facial
3. Mental
4. Pectoral
5. Axillary
6. Brachial
7. Antecubital or cubital
8. Carpal
9. Digital or phalangeal
10. Femoral
11. Patellar
12. Tarsal
13. Digital or phalangeal
14. Orbital
15. Buccal
16. Nasal
17. Oral
18. Sternal
19. Umbilical
20. Coxal
21. Inguinal
22. Pubic
23. Tibial
24. Dorsal

Figure 1.2, p. 3
1. Occipital
2. Cervical
3. Scapular
4. Vertebral
5. Olecranal
6. Sacral
7. Gluteal
8. Popliteal
9. Sural
10. Plantar
11. Calcaneal
12. Cephalic
13. Acromial
14. Dorsal

Figure 1.3, p. 4
1. Superior
2. Posterior
3. Anterior
4. Inferior

Figure 1.4, p. 4
1. Lateral
2. Medial
3. Proximal
4. Distal

Fill in the Blanks, p. 4
1. Superior
2. Lateral
3. Inferior
4. Distal
5. Anterior
6. Superior
7. superior
8. Proximal
9. Medial
10. Posterior

Identify Planes and Movements

Fill in the Blanks, p. 5
1. Frontal
2. Sagittal
3. Transverse
4. Abducts and adducts
5. Flexes and extends
6. Rotates

Identify Tissues and Their Functions

Figure 1.5, p. 5
1. Muscle
2. Epithelial
3. Nervous
4. Connective

Matching, p. 6
1. B
2. A
3. D
4. C

Fill in the Blanks, p. 6
1. Connective
2. Connective
3. Epithelial
4. Muscle and epithelial
5. Connective
6. Connective
7. Connective
8. Nervous

Describe Structures Involved in Movement

Functions and Properties of Structures, p. 6

1. Bone

Functions: provides framework and system of levers, protects underlying structures, stores minerals, and site forms blood cell formation (hematopoiesis)

Properties: firm, maintains constant shape

2. Ligament

Functions: connects bones to each other, limits motion, stabilizes joints

Properties: gristly texture, located between bones, maintains constant shape

3. Muscle

Functions: provides movement

Properties: corrugated texture, distinct fiber arrangements/directions, changes shape with movement

4. Tendon

Functions: protects, binds, and separates structures

Properties: wavy, dense, or smooth texture; connects all structures; becomes more pliable when heated or when tension is applied

Identify Special Structures

Figure 1.6, p. 6

1. Epidermis
2. Dermis
3. Superficial fascia
4. Blood vessels
5. Hair shaft
6. Nerve
7. Muscle

Figure 1.7, p. 7

1. External jugular vein
2. Subclavian vein
3. Superior vena cava
4. Axillary vein
5. Cephalic vein
6. Brachial vein
7. Inferior vena cava
8. Common iliac vein
9. Great saphenous vein
10. Femoral vein
11. Popliteal vein
12. Anterior tibial vein
13. Common carotid artery
14. Subclavian artery
15. Brachiocephalic artery
16. Axillary artery
17. Brachial artery
18. Heart
19. Abdominal aorta
20. Radial artery
21. Ulnar artery
22. Common iliac artery

23. Femoral artery
24. Popliteal artery
25. Posterior tibial artery
26. Anterior tibial artery

Figure 1.8, p. 8

1. Cervical lymph nodes
2. Right lymphatic duct
3. Axillary lymph nodes
4. Iliac lymph nodes
5. Inguinal lymph nodes
6. Thymus
7. Heart
8. Thoracic duct
9. Spleen
10. Cisterna chyli
11. Popliteal lymph nodes

Figure 1.9, p. 9

1. Brachial plexus
2. Musculocutaneous nerve
3. Radial nerve
4. Median nerve
5. Ulnar nerve
6. Lateral femoral cutaneous nerve
7. Common peroneal nerve
8. Brain
9. Cerebellum
10. Cervical plexus
11. Spinal cord
12. Intercostal nerves
13. Lumbar plexus
14. Sacral plexus
15. Sciatic nerve
16. Saphenous nerve
17. Tibial nerve

Figure 1.10, p. 10

1. Dendrites
2. Cell body
3. Muscle
4. Nucleus
5. Axon

Matching, p. 10

1. F
2. B
3. D
4. G
5. A
6. C
7. E

Word Challenge, p. 11

1. F
2. H
3. J

4. A
5. E
6. B
7. I
8. C
9. G
10. D

CHAPTER 2

Identify the Functions of Bone

Fill in the Blanks, p. 13
1. Support and protection
2. Movement
3. Hematopoiesis
4. Storage of minerals and fats

Identify Structures in Bone Tissue

Figure 2.1, p. 13
1. Osteocyte
2. Canaliculi
3. Lacuna
4. Haversian canal
5. Spongy bone
6. Concentric lamellae
7. Haversian canal
8. Volkmann canal
9. Compact bone
10. Osteon
11. Periosteum

Matching, p. 14
1. C
2. A
3. D
4. F
5. H
6. E
7. B
8. G

Identify Bones of the Human Skeleton

Figure 2.2, p. 15
1. Clavicle
2. Scapula
3. Humerus
4. Ulna
5. Radius
6. Carpals
7. Metacarpals
8. Phalanges
9. Hip (coxal) bone
10. Femur
11. Patella
12. Tibia
13. Fibula
14. Tarsals
15. Metatarsals
16. Phalanges
17. Cranium
18. Face
19. Sternum
20. Ribs
21. Vertebrae
22. Sacrum
23. Coccyx

Identify Shapes of Bones

Figure 2.3, p. 16
1. Long
2. Short
3. Irregular
4. Flat
5. Sesamoid

Classify Bony Landmarks

Functions of Structures
1. Depression
Function: houses muscles, tendons, vessels, or nerves
2. Opening
Function: allows passage of nerves, vessels, muscles, or tendons
3. Projection
Function: bumps that form joints
4. Attachment site
Function: bumps or ridges where tendons or ligaments attach

Matching
1. P
2. A
3. A
4. P
5. D
6. O
7. D
8. D
9. P
10. A
11. O
12. A
13. P
14. P
15. O
16. A
17. A
18. A
19. A

Identify Joints

Fill in the Blanks, p. 17
1. Joints are named according to the bones that articulate to form them.
2. Humeroulnar joint
3. The naming rule is modified by using the specific articulating bony prominence if a bone forms more than one joint.
4. Glenohumeral joint

Identify Joint Types
1. Synovial
2. Synovial
3. Synovial
4. Synovial
5. Synovial
6. Synovial
7. Cartilaginous
8. Synovial
9. Cartilaginous
10. Synovial
11. Synovial
12. Synovial
13. Fibrous
14. Synovial
15. Synovial
16. Synovial
17. Fibrous

Classify and Describe Synovial Joints

Figure 2.4, p. 18
A. 1. Ball and socket
   2. Triaxial
B. 1. Hinge
   2. Uniaxial
C. 1. Pivot
   2. Uniaxial
D. 1. Condyloid (ellipsoid)
   2. Biaxial
E. 1. Saddle
   2. Biaxial
F. 1. Gliding
   2. Nonaxial

Define and Identify Accessory Motions

Fill in the Blanks, p. 19
1. Optimal joint position
2. Compression
3. Loss of contact

Matching, p. 19
1. P
2. P
3. P
4. P
5. P
6. P
7. P
8. A
9. P
10. P
11. A
12. A
13. P

Word Challenge, p. 20
ACROSS:
1. meatus
4. trochanter
7. bone
8. spongy
10. crest
12. osteon
13. ulna

DOWN:
2. accessory
3. spin
5. rib
6. head
8. suture
9. nerve
11. tibia

CHAPTER 3

Compare Types of Muscle Tissue

Fill in the Blanks, p. 22
1. *Smooth:* involuntary, nonstriated, slow, steady contraction
2. *Cardiac:* involuntary, striated, moderate, strong contraction
3. *Skeletal:* voluntary, striated, short, strong contraction

Identify Skeletal Muscle Functions

Fill in the Blanks, p. 22
1. Movement
2. Posture
3. Protection
4. Thermogenesis
5. Vascular pump

Identify Fiber Arrangements

Figure 3.1, p. 23
A. Fusiform
B. Circular
C. Triangular
D. Unipennate
E. Bipennate
F. Multipennate

Matching, p. 23

1. F
2. E
3. B
4. A
5. C
6. D

Practice Naming Muscles

Fill in the Blanks, p. 24

1. Number of heads, location
2. Location, size
3. Size, location
4. Fiber direction, location
5. Action, size
6. Action
7. Shape, size
8. Shape, location
9. Action, shape
10. Location, fiber direction
11. Action, size
12. Location
13. Location
14. Shape, location
15. Location

Identify Skeletal Muscle Properties

Matching, p. 24

1. A
2. D
3. C
4. B
5. E

Identify Skeletal Muscle Structures

Figure 3.2, p. 25

1. Epimysium
2. Perimysium
3. Endomysium
4. Fascicle
5. Sarcoplasm
6. Single muscle fiber
7. Bone
8. Musculotendinous junction
9. Muscle belly
10. Nuclei
11. Sarcolemma
12. Z line
13. I band
14. A band
15. Mitochondria
16. Myofibril
17. Sarcolemma
18. Transverse tubule
19. Sarcoplasmic reticulum
20. Nucleus

Matching, p. 26

1. H
2. K
3. G
4. O
5. M
6. N
7. A
8. F
9. Q
10. D
11. L
12. B
13. P
14. I
15. E
16. J
17. R
18. C

Identify Structures and Events in Muscle Contraction

Figure 3.3, p. 27

1. Tropomyosin
2. Actin
3. Myosin head
4. Troponin
5. Crossbridge
6. Exposed binding sites

Order Skeletal Muscle Contraction Events, p. 27

_7_ Calcium ions bind to troponin.

_5_ Action potential travels down the transverse tubules to the sarcoplasmic reticulum.

_2_ Acetylcholine is released from the synaptic vesicles.

_9_ Cross-bridges form between actin and myosin.

_1_ Action potential travels down the axon of a motor neuron.

_10_ Power stroke occurs, pulling the sarcomere together.

_8_ Tropomyosin distorts, exposing binding sites on actin.

_3_ Acetylcholine molecules bind to receptors on the sarcolemma.

_6_ Calcium ions are released from the sarcoplasmic reticulum into the sarcoplasm.

_4_ Action potential initiated on muscle cell membrane.

Compare Skeletal Muscle Fiber Types

Matching, p. 28

1. IM
2. FT
3. ST
4. FT
5. IM
6. ST
7. ST
8. FT
9. FT
10. ST

Matching, p. 28
1. ST
2. ST
3. ST
4. FT
5. FT
6. ST
7. FT
8. FT
9. FT
10. FT

Types of Muscle Contractions

Figure 3.4, p. 28
1. Isometric
2. Concentric
3. Eccentric

Fill in the Blanks, p. 29
1. *Isometric:* stabilizes joints, maintains posture, resists against immovable objects
2. *Concentric:* initiates or accelerates movement, overcomes external resistance
3. *Eccentric:* decelerates or controls movements

Experience Different Types of Muscle Contractions, p. 29
1. *Raising arm:* deltoid shortens and becomes thicker and firmer, exaggerated when resistance (book) is added
2. *Holding arm out:* deltoid remains thick and firm and muscle fatigues over time
3. *Lowering arm:* deltoid continues to activate as it lengthens

Define Muscle Relationships

Definitions, p. 30
1. *Agonist:* most involved in joint motion and point of reference when describing muscle relationships
2. *Synergist:* assists other muscles or muscle groups by stabilizing, steering, or contributing a particular joint movement
3. *Antagonist:* performs opposite action or actions to agonist, essential to balanced posture and controlling movements

Matching, p. 30
1. A
2. B
3. E
4. D
5. F
6. C
7. I
8. H
9. G

Identify Muscles of the Human Body

Figure 3.5, p. 31
1. Orbicularis oculi
2. Masseter
3. Sternocleidomastoid
4. Deltoid
5. Pectoralis major
6. Serratus anterior
7. Biceps brachii
8. Brachioradialis
9. Flexor carpi
10. Extensor carpi
11. Adductors of the thigh
12. Peroneus longus
13. Tibialis anterior
14. Temporalis
15. Orbicularis oris
16. Trapezius
17. External oblique
18. Intercostals
19. Internal oblique
20. Rectus abdominis
21. Sartorius
22. Quadriceps femoris
23. Gastrocnemius
24. Soleus

Figure 3.6, p. 32
1. Teres minor
2. Teres major
3. Latissimus dorsi
4. Gluteus maximus
5. Biceps femoris
6. Semitendinosus
7. Semimembranosus
8. Gastrocnemius
9. Sternocleidomastoid
10. Trapezius
11. Deltoid
12. Triceps brachii
13. Gluteus medius
14. Peroneus longus

Classify Levers

Define the Components of a Lever, p. 33
1. *Axis/fulcrum:* part that the lever turns around (joints)
2. *Force:* internal source of mechanical energy (muscles)
3. *Resistance:* external source of mechanical energy (gravity, friction)

Types of Levers, p. 33
1. *First-class lever:* teeter-totter, atlanto-occipital joint, balance
2. *Second-class lever:* wheelbarrow, talocrural joint, power
3. *Third-class lever:* shovel, humeroulnar joint, speed and range of motion

Classify Proprioceptors

Matching, p. 34
1. E
2. B
3. D
4. C
5. A

Matching, p. 35

Structure	Stimulus or Trigger	Response to Trigger
Golgi tendon organ	Rapid change in muscle length	Contracts muscle
Muscle spindle	Excessive muscle contraction	Inhibits muscle contraction
Pacinian corpuscle	Vibration and deep pressure	Indicates direction and speed of movement
Ruffini ending	Distortion of joint capsule	Indicates position of joint
Vestibular apparatus	Change in head position	Re-establishes equilibrium

Range of Motion

Types of Range of Motion and Their Purpose
1. *Active range of motion (AROM):* determines willingness and ability to perform all voluntary movements at a joint
2. *Passive Range of Motion (PROM):* determines end feel and length of antagonist muscles
3. *Resisted Range of Motion (RROM):* determines strength and endurance of agonist and synergist muscles

Client and Practitioner Actions during Range of Motion
1. *Active range of motion (AROM):* client performs movement as practitioner observes
2. *Passive Range of Motion (PROM):* client relaxes as practitioner performs movement
3. *Resisted Range of Motion (RROM):* client performs as practitioner prevents movement

Word Challenge, p. 36
1. Proprioception
2. Agonist
3. Motor unit
4. Sarcoplasmic reticulum
5. Extensibility
6. Pennate
7. Synapse
8. Fast twitch
9. Isometric
10. Second-class lever
11. Inner ear
12. End feel
13. Aerobic
14. Actin
15. Fascicle

CHAPTER 4

Label Surface Landmarks

Figure 4.1, p. 39
1. Deltoid
2. Biceps brachii
3. Axilla
4. Pectoralis major
5. Serratus anterior
6. Clavicle
7. Sternum

Figure 4.2, p. 40
1. Acromion process
2. Deltoid
3. Triceps brachii
4. Clavicle
5. Sternum
6. Biceps brachii

Figure 4.3, p. 40
1. Upper trapezius
2. Superior angle of scapula

3. Lower trapezius
4. Biceps brachii
5. Triceps brachii
6. Deltoid
7. Spine of scapula
8. Lateral border of scapula
9. Medial border of scapula
10. Inferior angle of scapula
11. Latissimus dorsi

Color and Label Skeletal Structures

Figure 4.4, p. 41
1. Manubrium of sternum
2. Clavicle
3. Coracoid process
4. Acromioclavicular joint
5. Acromion process
6. Head of the humerus
7. Glenohumeral joint
8. Scapula
9. Sternoclavicular joint
10. Costocartilage
11. Body of sternum

Figure 4.5, p. 41
1. Clavicle
2. Acromion process
3. Head of humerus
4. Shaft of humerus
5. Supraspinous fossa
6. Spine of scapula
7. Infraspinous fossa

Match Muscles and Bony Landmarks

Matching, p. 42
1. P
2. D
3. E
4. H
5. B
6. O
7. A
8. N
9. K
10. M
11. C
12. J
13. Q
14. I
15. F
16. L
17. G

Label Joints and Ligaments

Figure 4.6, p. 42
1. Coracoclavicular ligaments
2. Acromion process
3. Coracoacromial ligament
4. Glenohumeral ligaments
5. Humerus
6. Clavicle
7. Sternoclavicular ligament
8. Sternum

Complete the Table: Ligaments, p. 43

Ligament	Bony Landmarks Joined	Function
Acromioclavicular	Lateral clavicle Acromion process	Anchors lateral clavicle to scapula, preventing elevation of lateral clavicle.
Coracoacromial	Coracoid process Acromion process	Stabilizes humeral head during overhead activities.
Coracoclavicular	Coracoid process Lateral clavicle	Prevents superior movement of lateral clavicle.
Coracohumeral	Coracoid process Humeral head	Stabilizes humeral head when arm is resting at the side.
Glenohumeral	Glenoid fossa Proximal humerus	Holds humeral head in glenoid fossa.
Sternoclavicular	Manubrium Medial clavicle	Anchors medial clavicle to manubrium of sternum.

Label Muscles of the Shoulder

Figure 4.7, p. 44
1. Trapezius
2. Deltoid
3. Pectoralis major
4. Coracobrachialis
5. Biceps brachii
6. Serratus anterior

Figure 4.8, p. 45
1. Trapezius
2. Deltoid
3. Infraspinatus
4. Teres minor
5. Teres major
6. Latissimus dorsi
7. Triceps brachii (long head)
8. Triceps brachii (lateral head)
9. Triceps brachii (medial head)

Figure 4.9, p. 45
1. Subclavius
2. Subscapularis
3. Teres minor
4. Coracobrachialis
5. Teres major
6. Pectoralis minor
7. Serratus anterior
8. Biceps brachii

Figure 4.10, p. 46
1. Levator scapula
2. Rhomboid
3. Supraspinatus
4. Infraspinatus
5. Teres minor
6. Teres major
7. Triceps brachii

Label Special Structures

Figure 4.11, p. 47
1. Deep cervical lymph nodes
2. Supraclavicular lymph nodes
3. Clavicle
4. Axillary lymph nodes
5. Pectoralis minor
6. Brachial artery
7. Brachial vein
8. Serratus anterior
9. Common carotid artery
10. Internal jugular vein
11. Subclavian artery and vein
12. Pectoralis major
13. Parasternal lymph nodes
14. Mammary tissue

Identify Shoulder Movements

Figure 4.12, p. 48
1. Elevation
2. Depression
3. Retraction
4. Protraction
5. Upward rotation
6. Downward rotation

Figure 4.13, p. 49–50
1. Flexion
2. Extension
3. Abduction
4. Adduction
5. Internal rotation
6. External rotation
7. Horizontal abduction
8. Horizontal adduction

Match Muscle Origins, Insertions, and Actions

Matching, p. 51
1. O
2. B
3. F
4. E
5. L
6. Q
7. G
8. J
9. K
10. I
11. A
12. M
13. P
14. C
15. N
16. H
17. D

Matching, p. 51
1. M
2. K
3. B
4. C
5. I
6. N
7. E
8. A
9. H
10. G
11. J
12. F
13. C
14. I
15. C
16. D
17. L

Matching, p. 52

1. L, O
2. L, O
3. K, M, N, O, P, Q, R
4. N, P
5. L, M, P, R
6. A, B, D, F, G
7. K, L, M, O, Q, R
8. E, H
9. F, G, I
10. E, H, J
11.
12. R
13. K
14. L, M, R
15. N, P
16. A, B, C, E, G, I, J
17. M

Identify Shortening and Lengthening Shoulder Muscles

Shortened and Lengthened Positions, p. 52

1. Latissimus Dorsi
Shortened position: shoulder extended, adducted, and internally rotated
Lengthened position: shoulder flexed, abducted, and externally rotated

2. Pectoralis Major
Shortened position: shoulder adducted and internally rotated
Lengthened position: shoulder abducted and externally rotated

3. Rhomboids
Shortened position: scapula elevated, retracted, and downwardly rotated
Lengthened position: scapula depressed, protracted, and upwardly rotated

4. Subscapularis
Shortened position: shoulder internally rotated
Lengthened position: shoulder externally rotated

5. Supraspinatus
Shortened position: shoulder abducted
Lengthened position: shoulder adducted

6. Teres Major
Shortened position: shoulder extended, adducted, and internally rotated
Lengthened position: shoulder flexed, abducted, and externally rotated

7. Triceps Brachii
Shortened position: shoulder extended and adducted, elbow extended
Lengthened position: shoulder flexed and abducted, elbow flexed

Complete the Table: Synergists/Antagonists

Complete the Table, p. 53–54

Movement	Muscles	Opposite Action
Scapular depression	Trapezius (lower fibers) Pectoralis minor Serratus anterior	Scapular elevation
Scapular downward rotation	Levator scapula Rhomboids	Scapular upward rotation
Scapular elevation	Trapezius (upper fibers) Levator scapula Rhomboids	Scapular depression
Scapular protraction	Pectoralis minor Serratus anterior	Scapular retraction
Scapular retraction	Trapezius (all fibers) Rhomboids	Scapular protraction
Scapular upward rotation	Trapezius (all fibers) Serratus anterior	Scapular downward rotation

Movement	Muscles	Opposite Action
Shoulder abduction	Deltoid (all fibers) Supraspinatus Pectoralis major (overhead)	Shoulder adduction
Shoulder adduction	Pectoralis major Latissimus dorsi Teres major Coracobrachialis Biceps brachii (short head) Triceps brachii (long head)	Shoulder abduction
Shoulder extension	Deltoid (posterior fibers) Latissimus dorsi Teres major Pectoralis major (costal fibers)	Shoulder flexion
Shoulder external rotation	Deltoid (posterior fibers) Infraspinatus Teres minor	Shoulder internal rotation
Shoulder flexion	Deltoid (anterior fibers) Pectoralis major (clavicular fibers) Coracobrachialis Biceps brachii	Shoulder extension
Shoulder horizontal abduction	Deltoid (posterior fibers) Infraspinatus Latissimus dorsi Teres minor	Shoulder horizontal adduction
Shoulder horizontal adduction	Pectoralis major Deltoid (anterior fibers)	Shoulder horizontal abduction
Shoulder internal rotation	Deltoid (anterior fibers) Pectoralis major Latissimus dorsi Teres major Subscapularis	Shoulder external rotation

Putting the Shoulder In Motion

Figure 4.15, p. 56

Reaching

1. **Joints:** shoulder, elbow, forearm, and wrist
2. **Shoulder movements:** shoulder flexion
3. **Sequence:** The shoulders flex as the elbows extend, placing the arms in position to intercept the ball as the hands clasp together.

Figure 4.16, p. 57

Rowing

1. **Joints:** ankles, knees, hips, trunk, shoulders, elbows, wrists
2. **Shoulder movements:** shoulder extension and horizontal abduction
3. **Sequence:** The driving force of the rowing motion occurs when the shoulders extend and horizontally abduct to pull the oar handles into the solar plexus.

Figure 4.17, p. 58

Casting a Line

1. **Joints:** shoulder, elbow, wrist
2. **Shoulder movements:** shoulder flexion followed by extension to cast the line forward
3. **Sequence:** The elbow and wrist remain relaxed and neutral as the shoulder first flexes raising the rod tip overhead then extends to cast the line forward.

Figure 4.18, p. 59

Drawing a Bow

1. **Joints:** scapula, shoulder, elbow
2. **Shoulder movements** (right-handed draw): scapular retraction and shoulder horizontal abduction
3. **Sequence:** Powerful scapular retraction begins the motion, followed by simultaneous shoulder horizontal abduction and elbow flexion.

Word Challenge, p. 60

1. Humerus: C
2. Manubrium: F
3. Teres minor: I
4. Scapula: G
5. Subacromial bursa: H
6. Deltoid: B
7. Trapezius: J
8. Axilla: E
9. Coracohumeral ligament: D
10. Brachial plexus: A

CHAPTER 5

Label Surface Landmarks

Figure 5.1, p. 62

1. Brachialis
2. Cubital fossa
3. Brachioradialis
4. Palmaris longus
5. Flexor carpi radialis
6. Radial styloid process
7. Olecranon process
8. Medial epicondyle
9. Flexor carpi ulnaris
10. Flexor tendons
11. Pisiform

Figure 5.2, p. 63

1. Olecranon process
2. Anconeus
3. Extensor carpi ulnaris
4. Ulnar styloid process
5. Lateral epicondyle
6. Brachioradialis
7. Extensor carpi radialis longus and brevis

8. Extensor digitorum
9. Radial styloid process

Figure 5.3, p. 64

1. Hypothenar eminence
2. Digital creases
3. Distal and proximal palmar creases
4. Thenar eminence
5. Distal wrist crease

Figure 5.4, p. 64

1. Interphalangeal joints
2. Metacarpophalangeal joints
3. Extensor pollicis longus
4. Anatomical snuffbox
5. Radiocarpal joint
6. Radial styloid process
7. Tendons of extensor digitorum
8. Ulnar styloid process

Identify Skeletal Structures

Figure 5.5, p. 65

1. Humerus
2. Lateral epicondyle
3. Radial head
4. Radial tuberosity
5. Radius
6. Radiocarpal joint
7. Medial epicondyle
8. Coronoid process
9. Ulna
10. Carpals
11. Metacarpals
12. Phalanges

Figure 5.6, p. 66

1. Olecranon fossa
2. Medial epicondyle
3. Olecranon of ulna
4. Ulnar styloid process
5. Carpals
6. Metacarpals
7. Phalanges
8. Lateral epicondyle
9. Radial head
10. Ulnar ridge
11. Lister tubercle
12. Radial styloid process

Figure 5.7, p. 67

1. Fifth distal phalange
2. Fifth middle phalange
3. Fifth proximal phalange
4. Fifth metacarpal
5. Capitate
6. Hamate

7. Pisiform
8. Triquetrum
9. Lunate
10. Ulnar styloid process
11. Ulna
12. First distal phalange
13. First proximal phalange
14. First metacarpal
15. Trapezoid
16. Trapezium
17. Scaphoid
18. Radial styloid process
19. Radius

Matching, p. 68
1. O
2. L
3. U
4. M
5. D
6. J
7. E
8. F
9. P
10. R
11. B
12. A
13. C
14. Q
15. H
16. T
17. G
18. K
19. I
20. N
21. S

Label Joints and Ligaments

Figure 5.8, p. 69
1. Humerus
2. Humeroulnar joint capsule
3. Radial collateral ligament
4. Annular ligament
5. Oblique cord
6. Radius
7. Medial epicondyle
8. Ulnar collateral ligament
9. Ulna
10. Interosseus membrane

Figure 5.9, p. 70
1. Olecranon fossa
2. Medial epicondyle
3. Olecranon process
4. Annular ligament
5. Ulnar ridge
6. Ulna
7. Lateral epicondyle
8. Radial collateral ligament
9. Radial head
10. Radius
11. Interosseus membrane

Figure 5.10, p. 70
1. Deep transverse metacarpal ligaments
2. Palmar metacarpal ligaments
3. Palmar carpometacarpal ligaments
4. Palmar ulnocarpal ligament
5. Palmar radioulnar ligament
6. Collateral ligaments
7. Joint capsule of first metacarpophalangeal joint
8. Joint capsule of first carpometacarpal joint
9. Palmar radiocarpal ligament

Complete the Table, p. 71

Ligament	Bony Landmarks Joined	Function
Annular	Radial head Proximal ulna	Stabilizes proximal radioulnar joint as forearm pronates and supinates
Collateral	Distal end of metacarpals Proximal, middle, and distal phalanges	Limits lateral movement of fingers
Deep transverse metacarpal	Distal ends of metacarpals 2–5	Limits finger abduction in phalanges 2–5
Interosseous membrane	Radius Ulna	Muscle attachment Limits lateral displacement between radius and ulna

Ligament	Bony Landmarks Joined	Function
Palmar carpometacarpal	Carpals Proximal ends of metacarpals	Stabilizes palm
Palmar metacarpal	Proximal ends of metacarpals	Limits abduction in fingers
Palmar radiocarpal	Distal radius Carpal bones	Stabilizes anterior wrist and palm
Palmar radioulnar	Distal radius Distal ulna	Stabilizes anterior wrist
Palmar ulnocarpal	Distal ulna Carpal bones	Stabilizes anterior wrist and palm
Radial collateral	Medial epicondyle Head of radius	Stabilizes humeroulnar joint and maintains position of radial head
Ulnar collateral	Lateral epicondyle Lateral edge of proximal ulna	Stabilizes humeroulnar joint and maintains position of olecranon

Label Muscles of the Elbow, Forearm, Wrist, and Hand

Figure 5.11, p. 72
1. Brachialis
2. Brachioradialis
3. Extensor carpi radialis longus
4. Extensor carpi radialis brevis
5. Flexor pollicis longus
6. Pronator quadratus
7. Biceps brachii
8. Brachialis
9. Pronator teres
10. Bicipital aponeurosis
11. Flexor carpi radialis
12. Palmaris longus
13. Flexor carpi ulnaris
14. Flexor digitorum superficialis
15. Flexor digitorum profundus
16. Flexor retinaculum
17. Palmar aponeurosis

Figure 5.12, p. 73
1. Triceps brachii (medial head)
2. Anconeus
3. Flexor carpi ulnaris
4. Extensor carpi ulnaris
5. Extensor digiti minimi
6. Extensor indicis
7. Triceps brachii (lateral head)
8. Brachioradialis

9. Extensor carpi radialis longus
10. Extensor carpi radialis brevis
11. Extensor digitorum
12. Abductor pollicis longus
13. Extensor pollicis brevis
14. Extensor pollicis longus

Figure 5.13, p. 74
1. Supinator
2. Flexor pollicis longus
3. Flexor digitorum profundus
4. Pronator quadratus
5. Lumbricals

Figure 5.14, p. 75
1. Extensor indicis
2. Anconeus
3. Supinator
4. Abductor pollicis longus
5. Extensor pollicis brevis
6. Extensor pollicis longus

Label Special Structures

Figure 5.15, p. 76
1. Cephalic vein
2. Medial cubital vein
3. Median nerve
4. Radial artery
5. Radial nerve
6. Cephalic vein

7. Brachial artery
8. Ulnar nerve
9. Medial epicondyle of humerus
10. Cubital lymph nodes
11. Basilic vein
12. Ulnar artery
13. Ulnar nerve
14. Palmar and digital arteries and nerves

Figure 5.16, p. 77

1. Ulnar nerve
2. Cubital notch
3. Posterior ulnar recurrent artery
4. Flexor carpi ulnaris
5. Extensor carpi ulnaris
6. Humerus
7. Radial nerve
8. Olecranon process
9. Anconeus
10. Recurrent interosseous artery

Figure 5.17, p. 78

1. Flexor retinaculum
2. Flexor retinaculum
3. Median nerve
4. Median nerve
5. Finger flexor tendons
6. Finger flexor tendons
7. Carpal bones

Figure 5.18, p. 78

1. Flexor tendons of the fingers and hand in synovial sheaths
2. Flexor digitorum superficialis and profundus in common flexor synovial sheath
3. Flexor pollicis longus
4. Flexor pollicis brevis
5. Abductor pollicis brevis
6. Flexor retinaculum
7. Flexor carpi radialis

Identify Movements of the Elbow, Forearm, Wrist, and Hand

Figure 5.19, p. 79

1. Elbow flexion
2. Elbow extension
3. Pronation
4. Supination

Figure 5.20, p. 79

1. Wrist flexion
2. Wrist extension
3. Radial deviation
4. Ulnar deviation

Figure 5.21, p. 80

1. Finger flexion
2. Finger extension

3. Finger adduction
4. Finger abduction

Figure 5.22, p. 81

1. Thumb flexion
2. Thumb extension
3. Thumb adduction
4. Thumb abduction
5. Thumb opposition
6. Thumb reposition

Matching, p. 82

1. L
2. N
3. Q
4. P
5. E
6. C
7. F
8. F
9. F
10. M
11. D
12. L
13. H
14. I
15. O
16. K
17. A
18. H
19. B
20. J
21. G

Matching, p. 83

1. C
2. N
3. U
4. O
5. H
6. F
7. I
8. J
9. Q
10. G
11. D
12. A
13. E
14. R
15. K
16. T
17. B
18. M
19. L
20. P
21. S

Matching, p. 83

1. H, J, L, Q
2. A
3. B
4. B, G, I
5. A, H, P
6. B, H, I, P
7. A, O, P
8. A, E, P
9. A, E, P
10. E, I, P
11. H, J, L
12. H, L, P
13. B, G, H, Q
14. B, O, Q
15. F, Q
16. B, F, Q
17. M, Q
18. B, Q
19. G
20. B, G
21. A, I

Identify Shortening and Lengthening Muscles

Shortened and Lengthened Positions, p. 84–85

1. Brachioradialis
Shortened position: elbow flexed
Lengthened position: elbow extended

2. Extensor Carpi Radialis Longus
Shortened position: elbow flexed, forearm supinated, wrist extended and radially deviated
Lengthened position: elbow extended, forearm pronated, wrist flexed and ulnar deviated

3. Extensor Carpi Ulnaris
Shortened position: elbow extended, wrist extended and ulnar deviated
Lengthened position: elbow flexed, wrist flexed and radially deviated

4. Extensor Digitorum
Shortened position: elbow extended, wrist extended, and fingers extended
Lengthened position: elbow flexed, wrist flexed, and fingers flexed

5. Flexor Carpi Radialis
Shortened position: elbow flexed, forearm pronated, and wrist flexed and radially deviated
Lengthened position: elbow extended, forearm supinated, and wrist extended and ulnar deviated

6. Flexor Carpi Ulnaris
Shortened position: elbow flexed, wrist flexed and ulnar deviated
Lengthened position: elbow extended, wrist extended and radially deviated

7. Flexor Digitorum Profundus
Shortened position: wrist flexed and fingers flexed
Lengthened position: wrist extended and fingers extended

8. Palmaris Longus
Shortened position: elbow flexed and wrist flexed
Lengthened position: elbow extended and wrist extended

9. Pronator Teres
Shortened position: elbow flexed and forearm pronated
Lengthened position: elbow extended and forearm supinated

Complete the Table: Synergists/Antagonists, p. 86–87

Movement	Muscles	Opposite Action
Elbow extension	Anconeus Extensor carpi ulnaris Extensor digiti minimi Extensor digitorum Supinator Triceps brachii	Elbow flexion
Elbow flexion	Biceps brachii Brachialis Brachioradialis Flexor carpi radialis Palmaris longus Flexor carpi ulnaris Pronator teres Extensor carpi radialis longus	Elbow extension

Movement	Muscles	Opposite Action
Finger abduction	Abductor digiti minimi Dorsal interossei	Finger adduction
Finger adduction	Palmar interossei	Finger abduction
Finger extension	Extensor digitorum Extensor indicis Extensor digiti minimi Interossei Lumbricals	Finger flexion
Finger flexion	Flexor digitorum superficialis Flexor digitorum profundus Flexor digiti minimi brevis Lumbricals Interossei	Finger extension
Pronation	Brachioradialis Flexor carpi radialis Pronator teres Pronator quadratus	Supination
Radial deviation	Flexor carpi radialis Extensor carpi radialis longus Extensor carpi radialis brevis Abductor pollicis longus Extensor pollicis brevis Extensor pollicis longus	Ulnar deviation
Supination	Biceps brachii Brachioradialis Supinator Extensor indicis Extensor carpi radialis longus	Pronation
Thumb abduction	Abductor pollicis longus Extensor pollicis brevis Flexor pollicis brevis Abductor pollicis brevis	Thumb adduction
Thumb adduction	Opponens pollicis Adductor pollicis	Thumb abduction
Thumb extension	Abductor pollicis longus Extensor pollicis brevis Extensor pollicis longus	Thumb flexion
Thumb flexion	Flexor pollicis longus Flexor pollicis brevis Opponens pollicis Adductor pollicis	Thumb extension

Movement	Muscles	Opposite Action
Thumb opposition	Opponens digiti minimi Opponens pollicis Flexor pollicis brevis Abductor pollicis brevis	Thumb reposition
Ulnar deviation	Flexor carpi ulnaris Extensor carpi ulnaris	Radial deviation
Wrist extension	Extensor carpi radialis longus Extensor carpi radialis brevis Extensor carpi ulnaris Extensor digitorum Extensor indicis Extensor digiti minimi Extensor pollicis longus	Wrist flexion
Wrist flexion	Flexor carpi radialis Palmaris longus Flexor carpi ulnaris Flexor digitorum superficialis Flexor digitorum profundus Flexor pollicis longus Abductor pollicis longus	Wrist extension

Putting the Elbow, Forearm, Wrist, and Hand in Motion

Figure 5.23, p. 88

Basketball Free Throw

1. **Joints:** shoulder, elbow, wrist, hips, knees, and ankles
2. **Elbow, wrist, and hand motions:** elbow extension and wrist flexion
3. **Sequence:** The elbow and the wrist extend to push the ball up and forward toward the basket until the ball rolls off the fingertips.

Figure 5.24, p. 89

Drawing a Bow

1. **Joints:** scapula, shoulder, elbow
2. **Elbow, wrist, and hand movements** (right-handed draw): elbow flexion
3. **Sequence:** Simultaneous shoulder horizontal abduction and elbow flexion complete the pulling motion once the scapula has initiated the motion by retracting.

Figure 5.25, p. 90

Casting a Line

1. **Joints:** shoulder, elbow, wrist
2. **Elbow, wrist, and hand movements:** elbow extension and wrist ulnar deviation

3. **Sequence:** Once the rod is fully forward, the elbow fully extends and the wrist ulnar deviates, whipping the line forward to place the fly. Some anglers use a rolling motion, accomplished by pronating the forearm, to avoid entangling with overhead brush.

Figure 5.26, p. 91

Tennis Backhand

1. **Joints:** scapula, shoulder, elbow, forearm, wrist, trunk, hips, knees
2. **Elbow, wrist, and hand movements** (right-handed swing): right elbow extension, right forearm supination, and right wrist extension
3. **Sequence:** The scapula retracts as the elbow extends, forearm supinates, and wrist extends to direct and place the shot.

Word Challenge, p. 92

ACROSS:

4. one
5. radius
7. ulna
10. brachioradialis
12. eight
14. oblique cord

DOWN:
1. anconeus
2. flexor carpi radialis
3. carpal tunnel
6. snuffbox
8. trapezoid
9. phalanges
11. supinate
13. hamate

CHAPTER 6

Label Surface Landmarks

Figure 6.1, p. 94
1. Supraorbital margin
2. Mental protuberance
3. Thyroid cartilage
4. Frontal eminence
5. Zygomatic bone
6. Mandible
7. Trapezius
8. Clavicle

Figure 6.2, p. 95
1. Nuchal ligament
2. Mastoid process
3. External occipital protuberance

Figure 6.3, p. 95
1. Temporal fossa
2. External occipital protuberance
3. Mastoid process
4. Thyroid cartilage
5. Trapezius
6. Clavicle
7. Posterior triangle
8. Angle of mandible
9. Mental protuberance
10. Anterior triangle
11. Sternocleidomastoid muscle

Color and Label Skeletal Structures

Figure 6.4, p. 96
1. Nasal bones
2. Sphenoid bone
3. Orbital cavity
4. Lacrimal bone
5. Ethmoid bone
6. Nasal cavity
7. Vomer
8. Mental protuberance
9. Frontal bone
10. Sutures
11. Parietal bones
12. Temporal bone

13. Greater wing of sphenoid bone
14. Zygomatic bone
15. Maxilla
16. Mandible

Figure 6.5, p. 97
1. Palatine process
2. Palatine bone
3. Sphenoid bone
4. Pterygoid plates
5. Styloid process
6. Temporal bone
7. Foramen magnum
8. Inferior nuchal line
9. Superior nuchal line
10. Occipital bone
11. Maxilla
12. Zygomatic bone
13. Vomer
14. Zygomatic process
15. Mandibular fossa
16. Basilar part of occipital bone
17. Occipital condyles
18. Parietal bone
19. External occipital protuberance

Matching, p. 98
1. F
2. I, N, R, S, W
3. E, F, I, J, L, M, P, Q, S
4. G, V
5. P
6. A, B, U
7. A, H, K
8. B, T
9. A, R, T
10. T
11. E, J, L, M, N, O, Q, R, W
12. G
13. V
14. G

Label Joints and Ligaments

Figure 6.6, p. 99
1. Alar ligaments
2. Cruciate ligament
3. Transverse ligament
4. Ligamenta flava
5. Atlas
6. Axis

Figure 6.7, p. 99
1. Tectorial membrane
2. Tectorial membrane (deep portions)
3. Occiput
4. Atlas
5. Axis
6. Posterior longitudinal ligament

Figure 6.8, p. 100
1. Ligamentum nuchae
2. Ligamenta flava
3. Interspinal ligaments

Figure 6.9, p. 100
1. Temporomandibular ligament
2. Stylomandibular ligament

Complete the Table, p. 101–102

Ligament	Bony Landmarks Joined	Function
Alar	Occiput Atlas	Limits rotation of atlanto-occipital joint
Anterior atlantoaxial	Atlas Axis	Stablizes atlantoaxial joint
Anterior atlanto-occipital	Occiput Atlas	Stabilizes atlanto-occipital joint
Anterior longitudinal	Anterior vertebral bodies	Stabilizes vertebral bodies during extension
Cruciate	Occiput Atlas	Limits vertical movement in the upper cervical vertebrae
Interspinal	Vertebral spinous processes	Limits movement between vertebrae during flexion
Ligamentum flavum	Vertebral laminae	Stabilizes cervical vertebrae and limits flexion
Ligamentum nuchae	Occiput Vertebral spinous processes	Muscle attachment site Stabilizes cervical vertebrae and limits flexion
Posterior atlantoaxial	Atlas Axis	Stabilizes atlantoaxial joint during flexion
Posterior atlanto-occipital	Occiput Atlas	Stabilizes atlanto-occipital joint during flexion
Posterior longitudinal	Posterior vertebral bodies Intervertebral disks	Limits flexion
Sphenomandibular	Sphenoid Interior surface of angle of mandible	Limits protraction and lateral movement of the mandible
Stylomandibular	Styloid process Angle of mandible	Limits anterior and lateral movement of the mandible

Ligament	Bony Landmarks Joined	Function
Tectorial	Anterior edge of foramen magnum Posterior longitudinal ligament	Stabilizes cervical vertebrae and limits flexion
Temporomandibular	Condyle of mandible Zygomatic process of temporal bone	Maintains position of temporomandibular joint
Transverse ligament of axis	Atlas Dens of axis	Maintains position of dens of axis against atlas

Label Muscles of the Head, Neck, and Face

Figure 6.10, p. 103
1. Sternocleidomastoid
2. Splenius capitis
3. Levator scapula
4. Anterior scalene
5. Middle scalene
6. Posterior scalene
7. Trapezius
8. Omohyoid

Figure 6.11, p. 104
1. Sternocleidomastoid
2. Trapezius
3. Semispinalis capitis
4. Splenium capitis
5. Splenius cervicis
6. Levator scapula

Figure 6.12, p. 105
1. Geniohyoid
2. Thyrohyoid
3. Omohyoid
4. Sternothyroid
5. Digastric
6. Mylohyoid
7. Stylohyoid
8. Digastric
9. Sternohyoid
10. Omohyoid
11. Sternocleidomastoid
12. Trapezius
13. Omohyoid

Figure 6.13, p. 105
1. Ligamentum nuchae
2. Splenius capitis
3. Splenius cervicis
4. Occiput
5. Semispinalis capitis
6. Middle scalene
7. Posterior scalene

Figure 6.14, p. 106
1. Longus capitis
2. Rectus capitis anterior
3. Rectus capitis lateralis
4. Longus colli

Figure 6.15, p. 106
1. Obliquus capitis superior
2. Rectus capitis posterior minor
3. Rectus capitis posterior major
4. Obliquus capitis inferior
5. Middle scalene
6. Posterior scalene
7. Semispinalis cervicis
8. Longissimus capitis
9. Rotatores (cervical)
10. Multifidi
11. Rotatores (thoracic)

Figure 6.16, p. 107
1. Temporalis
2. Orbital
3. Zygomaticus major and minor
4. Risorious
5. Galea aponeurotica
6. Frontalis
7. Procerus
8. Corrugator supercilii
9. Palpebral
10. Nasalis
11. Levator labii superioris
12. Buccinator
13. Obicularis oris
14. Masseter
15. Mentalis
16. Depressor labii inferioris
17. Depressor anguli oris
18. Platysma

Label Special Structures

Figure 6.17, p. 109
1. Frontalis muscle
2. Supraorbital nerve
3. Orbicularis oculi muscle
4. Supratrochlear nerve
5. Procerus muscle
6. Levator labii superioris muscle
7. Zygomaticus major muscle
8. Orbicularis oris muscle
9. Levator anguli oris muscle
10. Depressor anguli oris muscle
11. Depressor labii inferioris muscle
12. Mentalis muscle
13. Hyoid bone
14. External carotid artery
15. Thyrohyoid muscle
16. Omohyoid muscle
17. Thyroid cartilage
18. Sternohyoid muscle
19. Thyroid gland
20. Sternothyroid muscle
21. Sternocleidomastoid muscle (sternal head)
22. Sternocleidomastoid muscle (clavicular head)
23. Anterior scalene muscle
24. Facial nerve (zygomatic branch)
25. Facial nerve (temporal branches)
26. Parotid salivary gland
27. Facial nerve (buccal branch)
28. Facial vein
29. Facial nerve (mandibular branch)
30. Facial artery
31. Great auricular nerve
32. Lesser occipital nerve
33. Accessory nerve
34. Transverse colli nerve
35. Supraclavicular nerves
36. Levator scapulae muscle
37. External jugular vein
38. Trapezius muscle
39. Middle scalene muscle
40. Brachial plexus
41. Omohyoid muscle

Figure 6.18, p. 110
1. Buccinator muscle
2. Submandibular salivary gland
3. Hyoid bone
4. Thyrohyoid membrane
5. Thyroid cartilage
6. Thyroid gland
7. Esophagus
8. Trachea
9. Styloid process
10. Mastoid process
11. Sternocleidomastoid muscle

12. Internal carotid artery
13. External carotid artery
14. Internal jugular vein
15. Anterior scalene muscle
16. Middle scalene muscle
17. Posterior scalene muscle
18. Axillary artery
19. External jugular vein
20. Axillary vein

Figure 6.19, p. 111
1. Spinous process
2. Dura mater
3. Arachnoid
4. Pia mater
5. Superior articular facet
6. Vertebral veins
7. Vertebral artery
8. Vertebral body
9. Nucleus pulposus
10. Internal vertebral venous plexus
11. Spinal cord
12. Dorsal root of spinal nerve
13. Ventral root of spinal nerve
14. Spinal nerve roots
15. Posterior longitudinal ligament
16. Annulus fibrosus
17. Anterior longitudinal ligament

Outline and Label Borders of Caution Sites

Figure 6.20, p. 111
Refer to Figure 6.1C on page 189 in your textbook.

Identify Neck and Jaw Movements

Figure 6.21, p. 112
1. Cervical flexion
2. Cervical extension
3. Cervical lateral flexion: right
4. Cervical lateral flexion: left
5. Cervical rotation: right
6. Cervical rotation: left

Figure 6.22, p. 112
1. Temporomandibular elevation
2. Temporomandibular depression
3. Temporomandibular retraction
4. Temporomandibular protraction
5. Temporomandibular lateral deviation: right
6. Temporomandibular lateral deviation: left

Match Muscle Origins, Insertions, and Actions

Matching, p. 113
1. C
2. G
3. E

4. P
5. O
6. R
7. D
8. I
9. N
10. B
11. M
12. M
13. I
14. H
15. N
16. A
17. F
18. J
19. K
20. Q
21. L

Matching, p. 114

1. H
2. I
3. E
4. K
5. B
6. A
7. N
8. R
9. C
10. J
11. L
12. R
13. O
14. Q
15. G
16. D
17. P
18. S
19. M
20. H
21. F

Matching, p. 114

1. A
2. A, E, G
3. D, F
4. D, F, I
5. B
6. B, E, G
7. J
8. C, F
9. A

10. D, J
11. F
12. C, J
13. C
14. D, F, I
15. C, F, I
16. C, F, J
17. C, F, J
18. C, D, F, I
19. A
20. B, H

Identify Shortening and Lengthening Muscles

Shortened and Lengthened Positions, p. 115–116

1. Longus Colli
Shortened position: head and neck flexed, laterally flexed to same side, and rotated to the opposite side
Lengthened position: head and neck extended, laterally flexed to the opposite side, and rotated to the same side

2. Masseter
Shortened position: mandible elevated
Lengthened position: mandible depressed

3. Scalenes
Shortened position: head and neck flexed, laterally flexed to same side, and rotated to the opposite side with inhalation
Lengthened position: head and neck extended, laterally flexed to the opposite side, and rotated to the same side with exhalation

4. Semispinalis
Shortened position: head and neck extended, laterally flexed to same side, and rotated to the opposite side
Lengthened position: head and neck flexed, laterally flexed to the opposite side, and rotated to the same side

5. Splenius Capitis
Shortened position: head and neck extended, laterally flexed to same side, and rotated to the same side
Lengthened position: head and neck flexed, laterally flexed to the opposite side, and rotated to the opposite side

6. Sternocleidomastoid
Shortened position: head extended and neck flexed, laterally flexed to the same side, and rotated to the opposite side
Lengthened position: head flexed and neck extended, laterally flexed to the opposite side, and rotated to the same side

7. Temporalis
Shortened position: mandible elevated and retracted
Lengthened position: mandible depressed and protracted

Complete the Table: Synergists/Antagonists

Complete the Table, p. 116–117

Movement	Muscles	Opposite Action
Jaw depression	Suprahyoids Digastric Lateral pterygoid	Jaw elevation
Jaw elevation	Temporalis Masseter Medial pterygoid	Jaw depression
Jaw left lateral deviation	Left medial pterygoid Left lateral pterygoid	Jaw right lateral deviation
Jaw protraction	Medial pterygoid Lateral pterygoid	Jaw retraction
Jaw retraction	Temporalis	Jaw protraction
Jaw right lateral deviation	Right medial pterygoid Right lateral pterygoid	Jaw left lateral deviation
Neck extension	Sternocleidomastoid (upper cervicals only) Splenius capitis Splenius cervicis Semispinalis Rectus capitis posterior major Rectus capitis posterior minor Obliquus capitis superior Levator scapula Trapezius Rotatores Multifidi Semispinalis Interspinalis Iliocostalis Longissimus Spinalis	Neck flexion
Neck flexion	Sternocleidomastoid Platysma Longus colli Longus capitis Scalenes (anterior fibers) Rectus capitis anterior	Neck extension

Movement	Muscles	Opposite Action
Neck left lateral flexion	Left sternocleidomastoid Left scalenes Left longus colli Left splenius capitis Left splenius cervicis Left semispinalis Left obliquus capitis superior Left rectus capitis lateralis Left levator scapula Left trapezius Left intertransversarii Left longissimus	Neck right lateral flexion
Neck left rotation	Right sternocleidomastoid Right scalene Left longus colli Left longus capitis Left splenius capitis Left splenius cervicis Right semispinalis Left rectus capitis posterior major Left obliquus capitis inferior Left rectus capitis anterior Left levator scapula Right trapezius Right rotatores Right multifidi Right semispinalis	Neck right rotation
Neck right lateral flexion	Right sternocleidomastoid Right scalenes Right longus colli Right splenius capitis Right splenius cervicis Right semispinalis Right obliquus capitis superior Right rectus capitis lateralis Right levator scapula Right trapezius Right intertransversarii Right longissimus	Neck left lateral flexion

Movement	Muscles	Opposite Action
Neck right rotation	Left sternocleidomastoid Left scalene Right longus colli Right longus capitis Right splenius capitis Right splenius cervicis Left semispinalis Right rectus capitis posterior major Right obliquus capitis inferior Right rectus capitis anterior Right levator scapula Left trapezius Left rotatores Left multifidi Left semispinalis	Neck left rotation

Putting the Head, Neck, and Face in Motion

Figure 6.23, p. 118

Throwing

1. **Joints:** scapula, shoulder, elbow, forearm, wrist, neck, trunk, hips, knees, ankles
2. **Head and neck movements** (right-handed throw): neck right rotation
3. **Sequence:** The neck rotates right, keeping the eyes forward as the weight is transferred from the right leg to the left and trunk rotates left.

Figure 6.24, p. 119

Heading a Soccer Ball

1. **Joints:** head and neck
2. **Head and neck movements:** flexion and rotation of head and neck
3. **Sequence:** The head and neck flex once the ball strikes the forehead, driving the ball forward. Rotation of the upper neck directs the ball to the right or left.

Figure 6.25, p. 120

Swimming Crawl Stroke

1. **Joints:** shoulder, elbow, forearm, neck, trunk, hip, knee, ankle
2. **Head and neck movements:** *reaching* = neck right rotation, *pulling* = neck left rotation
3. **Sequence** (starting with right reach): The trunk and neck rotate fully right until the face is out of the water for breath. As the right arm transitions from reaching to pulling, the neck and trunk rotate left to neutral. Motion repeats on left, beginning with the trunk and neck rotating fully left until the face is out of the water for breath.

Figure 6.26, p. 121

High Jump

1. **Joints:** shoulders, neck, trunk, hips, knees, ankles
2. **Head and neck movements:** neck extension
3. **Sequence:** Following the running approach and jumping motion, the neck, trunk, and hips extend, creating "rolling" motion as the body clears the bar.

Word Challenge, p. 122

1. Digastric
2. Atlas
3. Axis
4. Mandibular fossa
5. Omohyoid
6. Risorius
7. Masseter
8. Occiput
9. Trapezius
10. Sternocleidomastoid
11. Lambda
12. Mandible
13. Trachea
14. Medial pterygoid
15. Zygomatic process
16. Maxilla
17. Dens
18. Lacrimal bone
19. Orbit
20. Thyroid cartilage

CHAPTER 7

Label Surface Landmarks

Figure 7.1, p. 125
1. Pectoralis major
2. Xiphoid process
3. Iliac crest
4. Umbilicus
5. Sternum
6. Rectus abdominis
7. Linea alba
8. Inguinal ligament

Figure 7.2, p. 126
1. Pectoralis major
2. Rectus abdominis
3. External oblique
4. Anterior superior iliac spine
5. Iliac crest

Figure 7.3, p. 126
1. Upper trapezius
2. Middle trapezius
3. Lower trapezius
4. Latissimus dorsi
5. Thoracolumbar aponeurosis
6. Scapula
7. Lamina groove
8. Posterior iliac crest
9. Sacrum

Color and Label Skeletal Structures

Figure 7.4, p. 127
1. True ribs
2. False ribs
3. Floating ribs
4. Sacroiliac joint
5. Costovertebral joints
6. Scapula
7. Spinous processes
8. Transverse processes
9. Ilium
10. Sacrum
11. Coccyx
12. Ischium
13. Pubis

Matching, p. 128
1. A, B, E, F, L, R
2. A, E, L
3. C, D, F, K
4. I
5. N, Q
6. A, B, C, D, E, F, I, J, O, P, R
7. D, I, J
8. J
9. G, J, M, N, O, P, Q
10. D, H, I, K, M, N
11. A, B, E, K
12. A, L

Label Joints and Ligaments

Figure 7.5, p. 129
1. Atlas
2. Axis
3. Thoracic curvature
4. Sacral curvature
5. Cervical curvature
6. Lumbar curvature

Figure 7.6, p. 130
1. Vertebral body
2. Superior articular facet
3. Transverse process
4. Lamina
5. Spinous process
6. Costal facet of transverse process
7. Inferior costal facet
8. Superior costal facet

Figure 7.7, p. 130
1. Vertebral foramen
2. Articular facet of the superior articular process
3. Lamina
4. Spinous process
5. Facet of the inferior articular process
6. Vertebral body
7. Transverse process

Figure 7.8, p. 131
1. Lumbosacral articular surface
2. Sacral promontory
3. Transverse ridges
4. Transverse process of first coccygeal vertebra
5. Coccygeal vertebrae
6. Superior articular process
7. Ala
8. Anterior sacral foramina
9. Apex
10. Coccyx

Figure 7.9, p. 131
1. Sacral canal
2. Facet of superior articular process
3. Ala
4. Posterior sacral foramina
5. Sacral cornu
6. Sacral spinous tubercles
7. Intermediate and lateral sacral crests
8. Median sacral crest
9. Sacral hiatus
10. Coccygeal cornu

Complete the Table: Ligaments

Complete the Table, p. 132

Ligament	Bony Landmarks Joined	Function
Anterior longitudinal	Occiput Anterior vertebral bodies Anterior sacrum	Limits extension of the vertebral column
Interspinous	Vertebral spinous processes	Limits spinal flexion
Intertransverse	Vertebral transverse processes	Limits spinal lateral flexion
Lateral costotransverse	Vertebral transverse processes Posterior rib facet	Stabilizes costovertebral joints
Ligamentum flavum	Vertebral foramen	Limits spinal flexion
Posterior longitudinal	Posterior vertebral bodies and intervertebral disks	Limits spinal flexion
Radiate	Vertebral bodies Posterior ribs	Stabilizes costovertebral joints Maintains rib position within rib cage
Superior costotransverse	Posterior rib Lamina of vertebra above	Stabilizes costovertebral joints
Supraspinous	Vertebral spinous processes	Limits spinal flexion

Label Muscles of the Trunk

Figure 7.10, p. 133
1. Sternocleidomastoid
2. Deltoid
3. Pectoralis major
4. Latissimus dorsi
5. Serratus anterior
6. External oblique
7. Abdominal fascia

Figure 7.11, p. 134
1. Trapezius
2. Latissimus dorsi

Figure 7.12, p. 135
1. Intercostals
2. Serratus anterior
3. Abdominal fascia
4. Internal obliques

Figure 7.13, p. 135
1. Rhomboid minor
2. Rhomboid major
3. Intercostals
4. External oblique

5. Longissimus
6. Spinalis
7. Longissimus
8. Iliocostalis
9. Thoracolumbar aponeurosis

Figure 7.14, p. 136
1. External intercostals
2. Internal intercostals
3. Pectoralis minor
4. Coracobrachialis
5. Serratus anterior
6. Rectus abdominis
7. Transverse abdominis

Figure 7.15, p. 136
1. Semispinalis capitis
2. Tendon
3. Levatores costarum
4. Semispinalis thoracis
5. Multifidus
6. Intertransversarii cervicis
7. Rotatores thoracis
8. Intertransversarii

Figure 7.16, p. 137

1. Sternocleidomastoid
2. Scalenes
3. Serratus anterior
4. External intercostals
5. Diaphragm
6. Rectus abdominis
7. Internal intercostals
8. Transverse thoracis
9. External oblique
10. Internal oblique

Label Special Structures

Figure 7.17, p. 138

1. Diaphragm
2. Liver
3. Gallbladder
4. Stomach
5. Colon
6. Lungs
7. Heart
8. Spleen
9. Pancreas
10. Small intestine
11. Bladder

Figure 7.18, p. 139

1. Diaphragm (left dome)
2. Spleen
3. Left kidney
4. Pancreas (outline)
5. Descending colon
6. Small intestine
7. Right lung
8. Liver
9. Right adrenal gland
10. Right kidney
11. Ascending colon
12. Appendix
13. Bladder

Figure 7.19, p. 140

1. Right lymphatic duct
2. Thoracic duct
3. Left internal jugular vein
4. Left subclavian vein
5. Cisterna chyli

Figure 7.20, p. 140

1. Superior vena cava
2. Inferior vena cava
3. Superior mesenteric artery
4. Femoral veins
5. Left subclavian artery
6. Left subclavian vein
7. Aortic arch
8. Cardiac vein
9. Coronary artery

10. Aorta
11. Kidney
12. Renal artery
13. Renal vein
14. External iliac arteries

Figure 7.21, p. 141

1. Splanchnic nerves
2. Hepatic plexus
3. Lumbar plexus
4. Sacral plexus
5. Superior gluteal nerve
6. Inferior gluteal nerve
7. Sciatic nerve

Figure 7.22, p. 142

1. First cervical spinal nerve
2. Pedicle of cervical vertebra
3. T5 spinal nerve
4. Lumbar enlargement of spinal cord
5. First lumbar spinal nerve
6. Cauda equina
7. Cervical enlargement of spinal cord
8. C8 spinal nerve
9. Intercostal nerves
10. External intercostal muscle
11. Transverse abdominal muscle
12. Psoas major muscle

Identify Trunk Movements

Figure 7.23, p. 143

1. Trunk flexion
2. Trunk extension
3. Trunk lateral flexion: right
4. Trunk lateral flexion: left
5. Trunk rotation: right
6. Trunk rotation: left

Figure 7.24, p. 144

1. Inhalation
2. Exhalation

Match Muscle Origins, Insertions, and Actions

Matching, p. 144

1. D
2. E
3. B
4. G
5. C
6. M
7. L
8. P
9. N
10. Q
11. F
12. H
13. P
14. O

15. K
16. I
17. J
18. A

Matching, p. 145
1. D
2. Q
3. B
4. O
5. F
6. C
7. J
8. M
9. N
10. I
11. P
12. E
13. J
14. L
15. H
16. G
17. K
18. A

Matching, p. 145
1. D
2. D
3. C, E, F
4. B, E
5. A
6. C, E, G
7. B
8. E
9. B, E, G
10. B, F
11. B, D, E
12. C, E
13. B, F
14. B, F

15. A
16. D
17. B, G
18. A

Identify Shortening and Lengthening Trunk Muscles

Shortened and Lengthened Positions, p. 146

1. Erector Spinae Group
Shortened position: trunk extended and laterally flexed to the same side and head and neck rotated to the same side
Lengthened position: trunk flexed and laterally flexed to the opposite side and head and neck rotated to the opposite side

2. External Oblique
Shortened position: flexed, laterally flexed to the same side, and rotated to the opposite side
Lengthened position: extended, laterally flexed to the opposite side, and rotated to the same side

3. Internal Oblique
Shortened position: flexed and laterally flexed and rotated to the same side
Lengthened position: extended and laterally flexed and rotated to the opposite side

4. Quadratus Lumborum
Shortened position: extended and laterally flexed to the same side while inhaling
Lengthened position: flexed and laterally flexed to the opposite side while exhaling

5. Rectus Abdominis
Shortened position: flexed and laterally flexed to the same side
Lengthened position: extended and laterally flexed to the opposite side

6. Semispinalis
Shortened position: extended and rotated to the opposite side
Lengthened position: flexed and rotated to the same side

Complete the Table: Synergists/Antagonists

Complete the Table, p. 146–147

Movement	Muscles	Opposite Action
Exhalation	External oblique Internal intercostals Internal oblique Rectus abdominis Serratus posterior inferior Subcostales Transverse abdominis Transverse thoracis	Inhalation

Movement	Muscles	Opposite Action
Inhalation	Diaphragm External intercostals Serratus posterior superior Levator costarum Quadratus lumborum Scalenes Pectoralis minor Serratus anterior	Exhalation
Trunk extension	Iliocostalis Longissimus Spinalis Quadratus lumborum Semispinalis Rotatores Multifidi Interspinalis	Trunk flexion
Trunk flexion	Rectus abdominis External oblique Internal oblique	Trunk extension
Trunk left lateral flexion	Left rectus abdominis Left external oblique Left internal oblique Left iliocostalis Left longissimus Left quadratus lumborum Left intertransversarii	Trunk right lateral flexion
Trunk left rotation	Right external oblique Left internal oblique Right semispinalis Right multifidi Right rotatores	Trunk right rotation
Trunk right lateral flexion	Right rectus abdominis Right external oblique Right internal oblique Right iliocostalis Right longissimus Right quadratus lumborum Right intertransversarii	Trunk left lateral flexion
Trunk right rotation	Left external oblique Right internal oblique Left semispinalis Left multifidi Left rotatores	Trunk left rotation

Putting the Trunk in Motion

Figure 7.25, p. 148
Shoveling
1. **Joints:** shoulders, elbows, wrists, trunk, hips, knees
2. **Trunk movements:** trunk extension
3. **Sequence:** Trunk, hip, and knee extension complete the shoveling motion that began in the shoulder and arm.

Figure 7.26, p. 149
Overhand Throw
1. **Joints:** scapula, shoulder, elbow, forearm, wrist, neck, trunk, hips, knees, ankles
2. **Trunk movements** (right-handed throw): trunk left rotation
3. **Sequence:** The left leg steps forward and trunk rotates left, beginning the throwing motion and generating force to be transferred to the right arm.

Figure 7.27, p. 150
Downhill Ski Turn

1. **Joints:** shoulders, trunk, hips, knees
2. **Trunk movements** (left turn): trunk rotation right
3. **Sequence:** The trunk rotates right, keeping the core pointed down the hill, as the hips extend and knees rotate, edging and maintaining parallel skis through the turn.

Figure 7.28, p. 151
Rowing
1. **Joints:** shoulders, elbows, wrists, trunk, hips, knees, ankles
2. **Trunk movements:** trunk extension
3. **Sequence:** As the oar drops into water, the leg and trunk extend to drive the "pull" of the rowing motion, followed quickly by the movements of the upper body.

Word Challenge, p. 152
1. Iliocostalis: F
2. Kidneys: B
3. Pedicle: G
4. Hepatic plexus: A
5. Twelve: C
6. Inhalation: J
7. Dura mater: D
8. Scoliosis: I
9. Diaphragm: E
10. Cauda equina: H

CHAPTER 8

Label Surface Landmarks

Figure 8.1, p. 154
1. Iliac crest
2. Femoral triangle
3. Tensor fascia latae
4. Rectus femoris
5. Vastus lateralis
6. Vastus medialis
7. Patella
8. Patellar tendon

Figure 8.2, p. 155
1. Gluteus medius
2. Gluteus maximus
3. Biceps femoris
4. Iliotibial band
5. Head of the fibula
6. Iliac crest
7. Tensor fascia latae
8. Greater trochanter of the femur
9. Rectus femoris
10. Vastus lateralis
11. Patella
12. Tibial tuberosity

Figure 8.3, p. 155
1. Adductor magnus
2. Semimembranosus
3. Semitendinosus
4. Gracilis
5. Pes anserine tendon
6. Gluteus medius
7. Gluteus maximus
8. Gluteal fold
9. Biceps femoris
10. Popliteal fossa

Color and Label Skeletal Structures

Figure 8.4, p. 156
1. Neck of femur
2. Ischium
3. Pubic symphysis
4. Patella
5. Medial femoral condyle
6. Lateral femoral condyle
7. Head of fibula
8. Fibula
9. Tibia
10. Iliac crest
11. Iliac fossa of ilium
12. Anterior superior iliac spine
13. Greater trochanter
14. Lesser trochanter
15. Shaft of femur
16. Patellofemoral joint
17. Tibiofemoral joint
18. Tibial tuberosity
19. Medial tibial condyle

Figure 8.5, p. 157
1. Fifth lumbar vertebra (L5)
2. Posterior superior iliac spine
3. Posterior inferior iliac spine

4. Coccyx
5. Ischial tuberosity
6. Shaft of femur
7. Medial femoral condyle
8. Medial tibial condyle
9. Sacroiliac joint
10. Ilium
11. Sacrum
12. Femoral head
13. Femoral neck
14. Greater trochanter
15. Lesser trochanter
16. Pectineal line
17. Intercondylar notch
18. Lateral femoral condyle
19. Lateral tibial condyle
20. Fibular head

Figure 8.6, p. 158
1. Posterior superior iliac spine
2. Sacrum
3. Posterior inferior iliac spine
4. Greater sciatic notch
5. Coccyx
6. Ischial spine
7. Lesser sciatic notch
8. Femoral head
9. Ischial tuberosity
10. Iliac crest
11. Anterior superior iliac spine
12. Anterior inferior iliac spine
13. Acetabulum
14. Superior ramus of pubis
15. Pubic tubercle
16. Inferior ramus of pubis
17. Greater trochanter
18. Femoral shaft

Matching, p. 159
1. F
2. E

3. C
4. I
5. E, G, H
6. B
7. H, I
8. J
9. D
10. A, B
11. F
12. C, I
13. G
14. F, H
15. B, G, H
16. E

Label Joints and Ligaments

Figure 8.7, p. 159
1. Iliofemoral ligament
2. Ischiofemoral ligament
3. Posterior sacrococcygeal ligament
4. Posterior sacroiliac ligaments
5. Sacrospinous ligament
6. Sacrotuberous ligament

Figure 8.8, p. 160
1. Medial meniscus
2. Medial collateral ligament
3. Tibia
4. Femur
5. Anterior cruciate ligament
6. Posterior cruciate ligament
7. Posterior meniscofemoral ligament
8. Lateral meniscus
9. Lateral collateral ligament
10. Proximal tibiofibular joint capsule
11. Fibula

Complete the Table: Ligaments

Complete the Table, p. 160–161

Ligament	Bony Landmarks Joined	Function
Anterior cruciate	Medial tibial plateau Posterior surface of lateral femoral condyle	Limits anterior glide of tibia and posterior glide of femur
Anterior sacrococcygeal	Inferior sacrum Anterior coccyx	Stabilizes sacrococcygeal joint

Ligament	Bony Landmarks Joined	Function
Anterior sacroiliac	Anterior sacrum Iliac fossa	Stabilizes sacroiliac joint
Iliofemoral	Inferior ilium Proximal femur	Limits hip extension and medial rotation
Iliolumbar	Anterior ilium Lumbar vertebral transverse processes	Stabilizes pelvic girdle
Inguinal	Pubis Anterior iliac spine	Muscle attachment site
Ischiofemoral	Posterior ischium Femoral neck	Limits hip medial rotation
Lateral collateral	Lateral femoral condyle Head of fibula	Limits lateral opening of the knee (varus deformity)
Medial collateral	Medial femoral condyle Medial tibial condyle	Limits medial opening of the knee (valgus stress)
Posterior cruciate	Posterior tibia Anterior surface of medial femoral condyle	Limits posterior glide of tibia and anterior glide of femur
Posterior meniscofemoral	Lateral meniscus Medial femoral condyle	Stabilizes lateral meniscus
Posterior sacrococcygeal	Inferior sacrum Posterior coccyx	Stabilizes sacrococcygeal joint
Posterior sacroiliac	Posterior ilium Posterior sacrum	Stabilizes sacroiliac joint
Proximal tibiofibular	Lateral tibial condyle Head of fibula	Anchors head of fibula and stabilizes tibiofibular joint
Pubofemoral	Superior ramus of pubis Anterior neck of femur	Limits hip abduction
Sacrospinous	Anterior sacrum Posterior inferior iliac spine	Stabilizes sacroiliac joint
Sacrotuberous	Posterior sacrum Posterior inferior iliac spine Ischial tuberosity	Stabilizes sacrum inferiorly Muscle attachment site

Label Muscles of the Pelvis, Thigh, and Knee

Figure 8.9, p. 162
1. Iliacus
2. Psoas
3. Tensor fascia latae
4. Sartorius
5. Pectineus
6. Adductor longus
7. Gracilis
8. Rectus femoris
9. Iliotibial band
10. Vastus lateralis
11. Vastus medialis

Figure 8.10, p. 163
1. Gluteus medius
2. Gluteus maximus
3. Vastus lateralis
4. Biceps femoris (long head)
5. Biceps femoris (short head)
6. Sartorius
7. Tensor fascia latae
8. Rectus femoris
9. Vastus lateralis
10. Iliotibial band

Figure 8.11, p. 163
1. Adductor magnus
2. Semitendinosus
3. Gracilis
4. Semimembranosus
5. Sartorius
6. Gluteus medius
7. Gluteus maximus
8. Iliotibial band
9. Biceps femoris (long head)
10. Biceps femoris (short head)
11. Popliteus

Figure 8.12, p. 164
1. Iliacus
2. Psoas
3. Pectineus
4. Adductor longus
5. Gracilis
6. Vastus lateralis
7. Vastus intermedius
8. Vastus medialis

Figure 8.13, p. 164
1. Gluteus medius
2. Gluteus minimus
3. Biceps femoris (long head)
4. Biceps femoris (short head)
5. Iliacus
6. Psoas
7. Rectus femoris
8. Vastus lateralis

Figure 8.14, p. 165
1. Gluteus medius
2. Gluteus minimus
3. Piriformis
4. Gemellus superior
5. Obturator internus
6. Gemellus inferior
7. Quadratus femoris
8. Semitendinosus
9. Biceps femoris (short head)

Label Special Structures

Figure 8.15, p. 166
1. Inguinal ligament
2. Superficial inguinal nodes
3. Femoral artery and vein
4. Deep subinguinal node
5. Superficial subinguinal nodes
6. Superficial lymphatic vessels
7. Great saphenous vein
8. Superficial inguinal nodes
9. Deep inguinal nodes
10. Deep lymph vessels
11. Femoral artery and vein
12. Femoral artery and vein and deep lymph vessels
13. Great saphenous vein
14. Popliteal nodes
15. Anterior tibial artery

Figure 8.16, p. 167
1. Lumbar plexus
2. Obturator nerve
3. Lateral femoral cutaneous nerve
4. Sacral plexus
5. Femoral nerve
6. Anterior cutaneous nerve
7. Inguinal ligament
8. Lateral branch of anterior cutaneous nerve
9. Medial branch of anterior cutaneous nerve
10. Rectus femoris muscle
11. Saphenous nerve
12. Common peroneal nerve
13. Superficial peroneal nerve
14. Deep peroneal nerve

Figure 8.17, p. 168
1. Superior cluneal nerves
2. Medial cluneal nerves
3. Inferior gluteal artery and nerves
4. Posterior cutaneous nerve
5. Medial circumflex femoral artery
6. Muscular branches of sciatic nerve
7. Semitendinosus muscle
8. Popliteal artery and vein
9. Tibial nerve
10. Medial sural cutaneous nerve
11. Small saphenous vein
12. Gluteus minimus muscle

13. Superior gluteal artery and nerve
14. Piriformis muscle
15. Sciatic nerve
16. First perforating artery
17. Second and third perforating arteries
18. Vastus lateralis muscle
19. Fourth perforating artery
20. Biceps femoris muscle (long head cut)
21. Common peroneal nerve
22. Lateral sural cutaneous nerve
23. Gastrocnemius muscle

Identify Hip and Knee Movements

Figure 8.18, p. 169
1. Hip flexion
2. Hip extension
3. Hip abduction
4. Hip adduction
5. Hip internal rotation
6. Hip external rotation

Figure 8.19, p. 169
1. Knee flexion
2. Knee extension
3. Knee internal rotation
4. Knee external rotation

Match Muscle Origins, Insertions, and Actions

Matching, p. 170
1. S
2. E
3. L
4. P
5. J
6. G
7. F
8. K
9. J
10. O
11. V
12. M
13. W
14. B
15. R
16. Q
17. O
18. A
19. D
20. O
21. O
22. H
23. C
24. U
25. I
26. N

Matching, p. 171
1. M
2. K
3. H
4. C
5. D
6. F
7. A
8. I
9. G
10. J
11. R
12. J
13. L
14. P
15. O
16. G
17. B
18. Q
19. I
20. N
21. I
22. J
23. E
24. Q
25. Q
26. Q

Matching, p. 172
1. B, D, E
2. B, E
3. B, C, E
4. C, D, H, I
5. A, B, C, D
6. A, C, D, E, F
7. A, E, F
8. B, E, I, J
9. D, E
10. A, D
11. D
12. A, D
13. B, E
14. A, D
15. I, J
16. D, E
17. D
18. E, G
19. A, D, E, I, J
20. C, F, I, J
21. C, F, I, J
22. A, D
23. A, E, F
24. G
25. G
26. G

Identify Shortening and Lengthening Pelvis, Thigh, and Knee Muscles

Shortened and Lengthened Positions

1. Adductor Longus and Pectineus
Shortened position: hip flexed and adducted
Lengthened position: hip extended and abducted

2. Adductor Magnus
Shortened position: hip adducted
Lengthened position: hip abducted

3. Biceps Femoris, Semimembranosis, and Semitendinosis
Shortened position: hip extended and knee flexed
Lengthened position: hip flexed and knee extended

4. Gluteus Maximus
Shortened position: hip extended and externally rotated
Lengthened position: hip flex edand internally rotated

5. Gluteus Medius and Minimus
Shortened position: hip abducted
Lengthened position: hip adducted

6. Gracilis
Shortened position: hip flexed and adducted and knee flexed and internally rotated
Lengthened position: hip extended and abducted and knee extended and externally rotated

7. Psoas and Iliacus
Shortened position: hip flexed and externally rotated
Lengthened position: hip extended and internally rotated

8. Rectus Femoris
Shortened position: hip flexed and extended
Lengthened position: hip extended and knee flexed

9. Sartorius
Shortened position: hip flexed, abductd, and externally rotated and knee flexed and internally rotated
Lengthened position: hip extended, adducted, and internally rotated and knee extended and laterally rotated

10. Tensor Fascia Latae
Shortened position: hip flexed, abducted, and internally rotated
Lengthened position: hip extended, adducted, and externally rotated

11. Vastus Medialis, Intermedius, and Lateralis
Shortened position: knee extended
Lengthened position: knee flexed

Complete the Table: Synergists/Antagonists

Complete the Table, p. 174–175

Movement	Muscles	Opposite Action
Hip abduction	Gluteus maximus (upper fibers) Gluteus medius Gluteus minimus Piriformis Sartorius Tensor fascia latae	Hip adduction
Hip adduction	Pectineus Adductor brevis Adductor longus Gracilis Adductor magnus Gluteus maximus (lower fibers)	Hip abduction
Hip extension	Adductor magnus (posterior fibers) Gluteus maximus Gluteus medius (posterior fibers) Biceps femoris (long head) Semimembranosis Semitendinosis	Hip flexion

Movement	Muscles	Opposite Action
Hip external rotation	Psoas Iliacus Sartorius Adductor brevis Gluteus maximus Gluteus medius (posterior fibers) Piriformis Gemellus superior Gemellus inferior Obturator internus Obturator externus Quadratus femoris Biceps femoris (long head)	Hip internal rotation
Hip flexion	Psoas Iliacus Sartorius Tensor fascia latae Rectus femoris Pectineus Adductor brevis Adductor longus Adductor magnus (anterior fibers) Gluteus medius (anterior fibers) Gluteus minimus	Hip extension
Hip internal rotation	Tensor fascia latae Gluteus medius (anterior fibers) Gluteus minimus Semimembranosis Semitendinosis	Hip external rotation
Knee extension	Rectus femoris Vastus lateralis Vastus intermedius Vastus medialis	Knee flexion
Knee external rotation	Biceps femoris	Knee internal rotation
Knee flexion	Sartorius Gracilis Biceps femoris Semimembranosis Semitendinosis Popliteus Gastrocnemius	Knee extension
Knee internal rotation	Gracilis Sartorius Semimembranosis Semitendinosis Popliteus	Knee external rotation

Putting the Pelvis, Thigh, and Knee in Motion

Figure 8.20, p. 176

Shotput

1. **Joints:** scapula, shoulder, elbow, wrist, head and neck, trunk, hips, knees, ankles
2. **Hip, thigh, and knee movements** (right-handed put): right hip and knee extension and medial rotation, left hip and knee extension and lateral rotation
3. **Sequence:** The hips and knees extend and rotate, turning the body toward the target.

Figure 8.21, p. 177

Kicking

1. **Joints:** trunk, hips, knees, ankles
2. **Hip, thigh, and knee motions** (left-footed kick): right hip and knee medial rotation, left hip flexion, and left knee extension
3. **Sequence:** Once the right foot is planted on the ground, the right hip and knee medially rotate as the left hip flexes and pulls the left leg forward. The left knee extends as the left foot makes contact with the ball.

Figure 8.22, p. 178

Downhill Skiing

1. **Joints:** shoulders, trunk, hips, knees
2. **Hip, thigh, and knee movements** (left turn): right hip extension and medial rotation, left hip extension and lateral rotation, right knee extension and medial rotation, left knee extension and lateral rotation
3. **Sequence:** The hips and knees first extend to "unweight" body then rotate, edging and maintaining parallel skis through the turn.

Figure 8.23, p. 179

Swinging a Bat

1. **Joints:** scapula, shoulder, elbow, wrist, neck, trunk, hips, knees
2. **Hip, thigh, and knee movements** (right-handed swing): right hip and knee medial rotation, left hip and knee lateral rotation
3. **Sequence:** Once a small step forward is taken with the left leg and the weight is spread evenly on both legs, the hips and knees rotate to "open" the hips forward. Rotation continues as trunk and arm motions complete the swing.

Word Challenge, p. 180

ACROSS:

1. pelvis
5. ilium
6. popliteus
8. knee
9. vastus
10. sciatic
12. femur
14. gemellus
15. genuvarum

DOWN:

1. pes anserine tendon
2. minimus
3. biceps femoris
4. gluteus maximus
6. psoas
7. sartorius
11. ASIS
12. patella
13. fibula

CHAPTER 9

Label Surface Landmarks

Figure 9.1, p. 182

1. Fibula
2. Peroneus longus
3. Extensor digitorum longus
4. Lateral malleolus
5. Tibialis anterior
6. Gastrocnemius
7. Soleus
8. Tibia
9. Medial malleolus
10. Tendon of anterior tibialis

Figure 9.2, p. 183

1. Head of fibula
2. Gastrocnemius
3. Soleus
4. Peroneus longus tendon
5. Achilles tendon
6. Extensor digitorum longus muscle
7. Peroneus longus muscle
8. Tibialis anterior
9. Extensor digitorum longus tendons

Figure 9.3, p. 184

1. Shaft of tibia
2. Extensor hallucis longus tendon
3. Gastrocnemius muscle (medial head)
4. Soleus
5. Achilles tendon
6. Calcaneus
7. Medial longitudinal arch

Figure 9.4, p. 184

1. Medial head of gastrocnemius
2. Medial edge of soleus
3. Medial malleolus
4. Lateral head of gastrocnemius
5. Lateral edge of soleus
6. Achilles tendon
7. Lateral malleolus
8. Calcaneus

Color and Label Skeletal Structures

Figure 9.5, p. 185
1. Lateral condyle of tibia
2. Proximal tibiofibular joint
3. Fibular head
4. Fibular shaft
5. Distal tibiofibular joint
6. Lateral malleolus
7. Calcaneus
8. Cuboid
9. Fifth metatarsal
10. Proximal phalanx
11. Middle phalanx
12. Distal phalanx
13. Medial condyle of tibia
14. Tibial tuberosity
15. Tibial shaft
16. Talocrural joint
17. Medial malleolus
18. Tarsals
19. First metatarsal

Figure 9.6, p. 186
1. Soleal line
2. Tibia
3. Medial malleolus
4. Subtalar joint
5. Talus
6. Navicular
7. Cuneiforms
8. Metatarsals
9. Proximal phalanx
10. Distal phalanx
11. Neck of fibula
12. Fibula
13. Lateral malleolus
14. Talus
15. Calcaneus
16. Cuboid
17. Middle phalanx

Figure 9.7, p. 187
1. Head (talus)
2. Neck (talus)
3. Body (talus)
4. Lateral tubercle of talus
5. Attachment of calcaneofibular ligament
6. Calcaneus
7. Peroneal tubercle
8. Cuboid
9. Navicular
10. Cuneiforms
11. Metatarsals
12. Phalanges
13. Tuberosity of fifth metatarsal

Matching, p. 188
1. A, B, H
2. F, H
3. E, I, J
4. L
5. G, L
6. B
7. D
8. G, K
9. G
10. F, G
11. I
12. A, K
13. K
14. L
15. L
16. L
17. A
18. C
19. D, J
20. E
21. E
22. C, L
23. J

Label Joints and Ligaments

Figure 9.8, p. 189
1. Talonavicular ligament
2. Anterior talofibular ligament
3. Anterior tibiofibular ligament
4. Posterior talofibular ligament
5. Calcaneofibular ligament
6. Calcaneocuboid ligament
7. Long plantar ligament
8. Bifurcate ligament
9. Dorsal cuneiform ligaments
10. Cuneometatarsal ligaments
11. Dorsal metatarsal ligaments
12. Tarsometatarsal ligaments

Figure 9.9, p. 189
1. Tibia
2. Anterior tibiotalar ligament
3. Tibionavicular ligament
4. Tibiocalcaneal ligament
5. Posterior tibiotalar ligament
6. Posterior talocalcaneal ligament
7. Calcaneus
8. Medial talocalcaneal ligament
9. Plantar calcaneonavicular ligament
10. Dorsal talonavicular ligament
11. Dorsal cuneonavicular ligaments
12. Dorsal tarsometatarsal ligaments

Complete the Table: Ligaments

Complete the Table, p. 190

Ligament	Bony Landmarks Joined	Function
Anterior talofibular	Distal fibula Lateral neck of talus	Limits forward glide of talus
Bifurcate	Calcaneus Cuboid Navicular	Limits inversion
Calcaneofibular	Medial calcaneus Distal fibula	Limits lateral motion of talocrural joint
Deltoid	Medial malleolus Talus Calcaneus Navicular	Limits medial motion of talocrural joint
Long plantar	Calcaneus Cuboid	Limits superior motion of cuboid
Medial talocalcaneal	Talus Calcaneus	Limits anterior motion of talus
Posterior inferior talofibular	Posterior talus Lateral malleolus	Stabilizes posterior ankle
Plantar calcaneonavicular ligament	Calcaneus Navicular	Supports medial arch of foot
Tibiofibular	Lateral distal tibia Lateral malleolus	Limits displacement between distal tibia and fibula

Label Muscles of Leg, Ankle, and Foot

Figure 9.10, p. 191
1. Peroneus longus
2. Tibialis anterior
3. Peroneus brevis
4. Extensor digitorum longus
5. Extensor hallucis longus
6. Gastrocnemius
7. Soleus

Figure 9.11, p. 192
1. Plantaris
2. Gastrocnemius
3. Soleus
4. Peroneus longus
5. Peroneus brevis
6. Abductor digiti minimi

7. Tibialis anterior
8. Extensor digitorum longus
9. Peroneus tertius
10. Extensor hallucis longus

Figure 9.12, p. 192
1. Extensor hallicus longus tendon
2. Tibialis anterior tendon
3. Gastrocnemius
4. Soleus muscle
5. Flexor hallicus longus tendon
6. Flexor digitorum longus tendon
7. Tibialis posterior tendon

Figure 9.13, p. 193
1. Tibialis posterior
2. Flexor digitorum longus
3. Popliteus muscle

4. Peroneus longus
5. Flexor hallucis longus
6. Peroneus brevis

Figure 9.14, p. 193

1. Flexor digitorum longus tendons
2. Flexor digiti minimi brevis muscle
3. Plantar interosseous muscle
4. Flexor digitorum brevis muscle
5. Abductor digiti minimi muscle
6. Calcaneus
7. Lumbrical muscles
8. Flexor hallucis brevis muscle
9. Flexor hallucis longus tendon
10. Abductor hallucis muscle
11. Plantar aponeurosis (cut)

Label Special Structures

Figure 9.15, p. 194

1. Deep lymph vessels
2. Popliteal nodes
3. Great saphenous vein
4. Posterior tibial node
5. Peroneal artery, veins, and lymph vessels
6. Small saphenous vein and lymph nodes
7. Posterior tibial artery, vein, and lymph vessels
8. Great saphenous vein
9. Anterior tibial node
10. Anterior tibial artery, vein, and lymph vessels
11. Dorsalis pedis artery, vein, and lymph vessels
12. Dorsal venous arch

Figure 9.16, p. 195

1. Popliteal artery and vein
2. Popliteal lymph nodes
3. Small saphenous vein
4. Common fibular (peroneal) nerve

Figure 9.17, p. 195

1. Superficial peroneal nerve
2. Deep peroneal nerve
3. Intermedial dorsal cutaneous branch of superficial peroneal nerve
4. Sural nerve
5. Anterior tibial artery
6. Saphenous nerve
7. Medial dorsal cutaneous branch of superficial peroneal nerve
8. Lateral branch of deep peroneal nerve

Figure 9.18, p. 196

1. Tibial nerve
2. Medial plantar nerve
3. Common peroneal nerve
4. Lateral plantar nerve

Identify Ankle and Foot Movements

Figure 9.19, p. 197

1. Ankle plantarflexion
2. Ankle dorsiflexion

Figure 9.20, p. 197

1. Foot inversion
2. Foot eversion
3. Toe flexion
4. Toe extension
5. Foot pronation
6. Foot supination

Match Muscle Origins, Insertions, and Actions

Matching, p. 198

1. F
2. I
3. J
4. D
5. K
6. B
7. H
8. A
9. C
10. L
11. E
12. G

Matching, p. 198

1. B
2. C
3. I
4. J
5. G
6. E
7. D
8. F
9. G
10. G
11. A
12. H

Matching, p. 199

1. B, D, F
2. B, C, F
3. A, C, E
4. A, C, E
5. A
6. A, D
7. A, D
8. B, D
9. A
10. A
11. B, C
12. A, C

Identify Shortening and Lengthening Leg, Ankle, and Foot Muscles

Shortened and Lengthened Positions, p. 199–200

1. Extensor Hallucis Longus
Shortened position: ankle dorsiflexd, foot inverted, and big toe extended
Lengthened position: ankle plantarflexed, foot everted, and big toe flexed

2. Flexor Digitorum Longus
Shortened position: ankle plantarflexed, foot inverted, and toes 2–5 flexed
Lengthened position: ankle dorsiflexed, foot everted, and toes 2–5 extended

3. Flexor Hallucis Longus
Shortened position: ankle plantarflexed, foot inverted, and big toe flexed
Lengthened position: ankle dorsiflexed, foot everted, and big toe extended

4. Gastrocnemius
Shortened position: knee flexed and ankle plantarflexed
Lengthened position: knee extended and ankle dorsiflexed

5. Peroneus Brevis
Shortened position: ankle plantarflexed and foot everted
Lengthened position: ankle dorsiflexed and foot inverted

6. Peroneus Longus
Shortened position: ankle plantarflexed and foot everted
Lengthened position: ankle dorsiflexed and foot inverted

7. Peroneus Tertius
Shortened position: ankle dorsiflexed and foot everted
Lengthened position: ankle plantarflexed and foot inverted

8. Plantaris
Shortened position: knee flexed and ankle plantarflexed
Lengthened position: knee extended and ankle dorsiflexed

9. Soleus
Shortened position: ankle plantarflexed
Lengthened position: ankle dorsiflexed

10. Tibialis Anterior
Shortened position: ankle dorsiflexed and foot inverted
Lengthened position: ankle plantarflexed and foot everted

11. Tibialis Posterior
Shortened position: ankle plantarflexed and foot inverted
Lengthened position: ankle dorsiflexed and foot everted

Complete the Table: Synergists/Antagonists

Complete the Table, p. 201

Movement	Muscles	Opposite Action
Dorsiflexion	Extensor digitorum longus Extensor hallucis longus Peroneus tertius Tibialis anterior	Plantarflexion
Eversion	Extensor digitorum longus Peroneus longus Peroneus brevis Peroneus tertius	Inversion
Inversion	Tibialis anterior Extensor hallucis longus Tibialis posterior Flexor digitorum longus Flexor hallucis longus	Eversion

Movement	Muscles	Opposite Action
Plantarflexion	Gastrocnemius Soleus Plantaris Peroneus longus Peroneus brevis Peroneus tertius Tibialis posterior Flexor digitorum longus Flexor hallucis longus	Dorsiflexion
Toe extension	Extensor digitorum longus Extensor hallucis longus	Toe flexion
Toe flexion	Flexor digitorum longus Flexor hallucis longus	Toe extension

Putting the Leg, Ankle, and Foot in Motion

Figure 9.21, p. 202

Throwing

1. **Joints:** scapula, shoulder, elbow, forearm, wrist, neck, trunk, hips, knees, ankles
2. **Movements** (right-handed throw): right ankle plantarflexion and left ankle dorsiflexion
3. **Sequence:** As the hips and knees lunge and rotate to "open" the pelvis, the left ankle dorsiflexes, pulling the body over the lead leg. The right ankle plantarflexes, driving the body forward from the trail leg.

Figure 9.22, p. 203

Swimming Flutter Kick

1. **Joints:** hip, knee, ankle
2. **Leg and foot movements:** alternating hip flexion, knee extension, ankle dorsiflexion
3. **Sequence**

Figure 9.23, p. 204

High Jump

1. **Joints:** shoulders, neck, trunk, hips, knees, ankles
2. **Leg and foot movements:** ankle plantarflexion
3. **Sequence:** Following the approach, the jumping motion is initiated by single-leg hip and knee extension and ankle plantarflexion.

Figure 9.24, p. 205

Karate Thrust Kick

1. **Joints:** neck, trunk, hips, knees, ankles
2. **Leg and foot movements** (right-footed kick): right ankle plantarflexion

3. **Sequence:** The left foot is planted and left hip abducts as knee remains extended, lowering the body into an L-shape between the trunk and left leg. The right ankle plantarflexes as the right hip and knee extend, thrusting the foot forward for contact.

Word Challenge, p. 206

1. Pes planus
2. Extensor hallucis longus
3. Soleus
4. Plantar flexion
5. Gait
6. Lumbricals
7. Talus
8. Phalanx
9. Gastrocnemius
10. Calcaneus
11. Medial malleolus
12. Talocrural
13. Tibia
14. Peroneus longus
15. Dorsal
16. Hallux
17. Fibula
18. Plantar aponeurosis
19. Popliteal artery
20. Tibial tuberosity